Independent RNC-MNN Study Guide 2027-2028:

750 Practice questions with Detailed Answer Explanation, Covering All Domains for the NCC Maternal Newborn Nursing Exam

Caldwell Abiodun

Author Introduction

Excellence in maternal and neonatal healthcare demands more than clinical experience—it requires validated expertise grounded in rigorous national standards. Certification through the National Certification Corporation (NCC) represents a commitment to professional distinction, evidence-based practice, and lifelong learning. This study guide has been developed with that level of commitment in mind.

The author of this guide is an experienced educator and subject-matter specialist who has dedicated years to preparing healthcare professionals for high-stakes certification examinations. Working in close collaboration with a team of practicing clinicians, academic instructors, and assessment consultants, the author brings together both frontline clinical insight and deep familiarity with competency-based testing frameworks. This combined expertise ensures that the material presented here reflects not only the published content outlines but also the practical reasoning skills required to succeed on NCC examinations.

Understanding that candidates pursuing NCC certification are often balancing demanding clinical roles with personal responsibilities, this guide is structured to maximize clarity, efficiency, and retention. Complex topics are distilled into focused explanations that emphasize core principles, clinical application, and critical thinking. Rather than overwhelming readers with excessive detail, the content prioritizes high-yield concepts, commonly tested scenarios, and areas where candidates historically encounter difficulty. Each section is intentionally aligned with the exam blueprint, reinforcing both knowledge mastery and confidence under timed conditions.

Beyond content review, this guide reflects a philosophy of preparation rooted in professional empowerment. Certification is not merely an academic milestone; it is a reflection of advanced competence and dedication to patient-centered care. The author and contributing team recognize the responsibility that accompanies this credential and have designed this resource to support candidates in demonstrating both intellectual readiness and clinical judgment.

Every chapter has undergone careful review to ensure accuracy, relevance, and alignment with current standards of practice. The collaborative process behind this guide mirrors the interdisciplinary nature of healthcare itself—bringing together diverse expertise with a shared goal: to equip candidates with the tools they need to perform at their highest level.

This study guide stands as both a comprehensive review and a strategic roadmap, created to support dedicated professionals as they pursue certification and continue advancing the quality of care they provide.

Table of Content

Disclaimer

Chapter 1 — Pregnancy, Birth Risk Factors, and Complications

Pregnancy represents a physiologic continuum marked by profound systemic changes. Within this period, maternal adaptation supports fetal growth while maintaining maternal equilibrium. The nursing role during this phase includes identifying risk factors, monitoring maternal-fetal wellbeing, and applying anticipatory guidance to prevent complications. According to the provided materials, nurses must understand reproductive physiology, hormonal modulation, and environmental influences that contribute to pregnancy outcomes.

Reproductive Physiology and Early Adaptation

The reproductive system undergoes structural and functional changes beginning with conception. The uterus expands through hypertrophy of myometrial fibers and increased vascularization. Cervical glands produce a mucus plug that forms a barrier against infection. The ovaries, influenced by human chorionic gonadotropin, sustain the corpus luteum to maintain progesterone secretion until placental autonomy develops.

Systemically, increased blood volume, cardiac output, and oxygen demand reflect the maternal body's capacity to sustain dual circulation. The respiratory system adapts through diaphragmatic elevation and heightened sensitivity to carbon dioxide, enhancing oxygen delivery to the fetus. Concurrently, renal plasma flow and glomerular filtration rate rise, supporting metabolic waste elimination for both mother and fetus.

Hormonal influences—primarily progesterone, estrogen, and relaxin—modulate these adaptations. Progesterone reduces uterine contractility and smooth muscle tone, preventing preterm labor, while estrogen promotes vascularization and ductal growth in breast tissue. Relaxin aids pelvic flexibility in preparation for birth. These coordinated mechanisms are essential for maintaining gestational homeostasis.

Risk Factors Influencing Pregnancy Outcomes

Risk recognition is central to prenatal and perinatal nursing practice. According to the Core Curriculum, key categories of risk include physiologic, genetic, behavioral, and environmental factors.

- *Physiologic risks* encompass hypertensive disorders, diabetes mellitus, cardiac disease, and thyroid imbalance.
- *Genetic factors* may influence chromosomal anomalies, congenital malformations, and inherited metabolic disorders.
- *Behavioral risks* include substance use, inadequate nutrition, and noncompliance with prenatal care.
- *Environmental influences* such as exposure to toxins, radiation, or infectious agents also elevate fetal and maternal risk.

Nurses perform early identification through comprehensive history-taking, risk screening, and interpretation of diagnostic data. For instance, elevated blood pressure before 20 weeks may indicate chronic hypertension, whereas onset after midpregnancy with proteinuria suggests preeclampsia. Similarly, abnormal glucose tolerance screening necessitates dietary counseling and medical management to prevent macrosomia and neonatal hypoglycemia.

Preventive strategies emphasize anticipatory education—teaching about nutrition, rest, warning signs of complications, and adherence to prenatal visits. Counseling on teratogenic avoidance, vaccination, and medication safety further supports positive outcomes. Effective communication ensures that culturally diverse families receive appropriate health information in understandable terms.

Common Complications During Pregnancy and Birth

The management of pregnancy complications integrates pathophysiologic knowledge with prompt clinical decision-making. **Hypertensive disorders**, including gestational hypertension, preeclampsia, and eclampsia, remain leading causes of maternal morbidity. The condition stems from abnormal placental perfusion and endothelial dysfunction, resulting in systemic vasospasm and organ hypoperfusion. Nursing care includes frequent blood pressure assessment, evaluation for proteinuria, and observation for neurologic symptoms such as headache or visual changes.

Hemorrhagic complications, notably placenta previa and placental abruption, demand vigilant surveillance. Placenta previa presents as painless vaginal bleeding from low placental implantation, whereas abruption manifests with abdominal pain, uterine rigidity, and potential fetal distress. Rapid response through oxygenation, intravenous access, and communication with the interdisciplinary team ensures maternal-fetal stabilization.

Preterm labor is another significant concern, often related to infection, cervical insufficiency, or uterine overdistension. Recognition of uterine contractions before 37 weeks, accompanied by cervical change, prompts early intervention. Management strategies may include hydration, rest, and pharmacologic tocolysis under provider direction.

In all cases, nursing priorities focus on **early detection, stabilization, and coordination of care**. Emotional support for families experiencing complicated pregnancies is essential. Patient teaching emphasizes the importance of self-monitoring for symptoms such as bleeding, headache, decreased fetal movement, or fluid leakage.

According to the provided material, consistent assessment and anticipatory education form the core of risk management during pregnancy and birth.

Chapter 2 — Maternal Postpartum Assessment, Management, and Education

The postpartum period, extending from delivery through the return of the reproductive system to its pre-pregnancy state, is a critical phase for maternal adaptation. Nursing practice during this period centers on assessment, prevention of complications, emotional support, and patient education. According to the provided material, postpartum recovery is influenced by physiologic involution, lactation processes, and psychosocial adaptation. Nurses guide patients through physical healing, self-care, and newborn integration while monitoring for early signs of deviation from normal recovery.

Physiologic Assessment of the Postpartum Patient

Immediately following delivery, maternal systems begin a process of rapid involution. The uterus contracts under the influence of oxytocin, reducing in size and descending into the pelvis. Fundal assessment remains a core nursing skill; the uterus should be firm, midline, and descending approximately one fingerbreadth per day. A soft or "boggy" fundus indicates uterine atony and possible hemorrhage.

The **lochia**—postpartum vaginal discharge—progresses from rubra (dark red) to serosa (pink or brown) to alba (white or yellow). Accurate documentation of color, amount, and odor assists in early detection of infection or abnormal bleeding. Perineal assessment includes inspection for lacerations, episiotomy healing, and signs of hematoma formation.

Systemically, nurses monitor for cardiovascular adaptation as blood volume redistributes, potentially leading to transient bradycardia. Hematologic changes include leukocytosis and mild diuresis as fluid balance normalizes. Breasts should be assessed for engorgement, nipple trauma, or signs of mastitis. Temperature elevation within 24 hours may reflect dehydration or breast engorgement, whereas sustained fever suggests infection.

Patient comfort and recovery depend on comprehensive assessment encompassing urinary output, bowel function, sleep, and pain control. Early ambulation supports circulation, decreases venous stasis, and promotes bowel motility, but safety precautions are essential to prevent falls during orthostatic shifts.

Nursing Management and Interventions

Evidence-based postpartum management integrates physiologic care with individualized teaching and psychosocial support. Nurses encourage **uterine contraction maintenance** through fundal massage and bladder emptying. Administration of oxytocin enhances uterine tone and minimizes hemorrhage risk. Adequate hydration, balanced nutrition, and rest support tissue recovery and milk production.

Pain management involves assessment of both perineal and incisional discomfort. For vaginal births, cold compresses and sitz baths relieve edema and promote healing. After cesarean birth, pain control through multimodal analgesia, early ambulation, and respiratory exercises prevents pulmonary complications.

Nurses also play a pivotal role in **lactation support**. According to the provided materials, patient education should include latch technique, frequency of feeding, and recognition of adequate infant intake. Non-breastfeeding patients benefit from guidance on breast binding or ice packs to suppress lactation.

Psychological well-being requires equal attention. Emotional lability is common due to hormonal fluctuation and fatigue. The nurse's supportive presence facilitates discussion of feelings, reinforces coping skills, and identifies potential mood disorders. Persistent sadness or detachment may signal postpartum depression, warranting referral and family education.

Teaching extends beyond hospital discharge, covering hygiene, nutrition, exercise, contraception, and signs requiring medical attention. Encouraging self-efficacy in newborn care—diapering, bathing, safe sleep positioning—enhances confidence and strengthens maternal-infant bonding.

Patient Education and Discharge Readiness

Effective discharge planning begins upon admission and continues throughout hospitalization. The nurse ensures the patient demonstrates understanding of self-care, medication schedules, and warning signs such as excessive bleeding, severe pain, fever, or leg swelling. According to the provided material, education should be interactive and culturally sensitive, allowing for demonstration and feedback.

Teaching priorities include:

- **Physical recovery:** Instruction on perineal care, wound observation, rest, and gradual resumption of activities.
- **Breast care:** Recognition of engorgement or infection and guidance for continued lactation or suppression.
- **Family adaptation:** Support for partner involvement and awareness of emotional transitions.
- **Safety:** Emphasis on proper infant positioning, car seat use, and avoidance of co-sleeping hazards.

Follow-up appointments are critical for monitoring healing, contraception planning, and addressing breastfeeding concerns. Nurses reinforce that healing extends beyond the physical dimension—emotional stability and confidence are integral indicators of postpartum wellness.

In conclusion, postpartum nursing care embodies a balance of **clinical vigilance and holistic teaching**. Continuous assessment, individualized care, and empathetic communication ensure that recovery transitions smoothly from hospital to home.

Maternal Education and Health Promotion

Education during the postpartum period extends beyond discharge instructions—it is a process of empowerment that strengthens maternal confidence and fosters family stability. According to the provided material, effective health teaching integrates physical, psychological, and social perspectives.

Nurses act as educators, advocates, and role models, helping new mothers navigate recovery while adapting to parenthood.

Topics include nutrition for recovery and lactation, contraceptive choices, hygiene, and rest. Diets rich in protein, calcium, and iron assist in tissue repair and prevent anemia. Adequate hydration supports milk production, and gradual physical activity helps restore muscle tone. Patients are encouraged to engage in pelvic floor exercises once cleared, promoting circulation and bladder control.

Education must address **contraception counseling**, emphasizing postpartum fertility variations. For lactating women, non-hormonal or progestin-only methods may be preferred to avoid interference with milk supply. Nurses clarify misconceptions and ensure understanding of initiation timing and safety precautions.

Health promotion also involves immunization reinforcement—rubella and Tdap vaccines are reviewed before discharge when indicated. Discussion of spacing between pregnancies reinforces maternal recovery and infant health. The nurse's proactive communication style ensures that teaching is patient-centered and culturally congruent.

Psychosocial Adaptation and Family Integration

Postpartum emotional adaptation progresses through predictable stages—taking in, taking hold, and letting go. In the **taking-in phase**, the mother is dependent, reflecting on the birth experience and needing physical care. The **taking-hold phase** marks increased attention to learning infant care and self-management. By the **letting-go phase**, the woman begins to redefine her role and integrate her maternal identity.

Supportive nursing care recognizes these stages and promotes confidence through positive reinforcement and active listening. The presence of a consistent, compassionate caregiver aids emotional stability and promotes trust. When mood disturbances extend beyond transient "baby blues," the nurse must assess for postpartum depression or anxiety and provide timely referral.

The partner and family also undergo transition. Fathers or partners may experience emotional strain or role uncertainty. Nursing interventions should include inclusive education and encouragement of involvement in newborn care. Family-centered teaching normalizes the adjustment process and emphasizes shared responsibility.

Social determinants such as financial stress, housing, and access to care can affect recovery. Connecting families to community resources—support groups, visiting nurse services, and nutritional programs—enhances long-term stability.

Case Integration Example

A 28-year-old woman, 24 hours post spontaneous vaginal delivery, reports dizziness and heavy bleeding. Assessment reveals a soft, displaced uterus with excessive lochia rubra. Immediate nursing intervention includes assisting her to void and performing fundal massage to promote contraction. Intravenous oxytocin is administered as prescribed. After stabilization, the nurse reviews bladder habits, uterine assessment, and warning signs of hemorrhage.

Later, during discharge teaching, the same patient expresses concern about emotional changes and exhaustion. The nurse provides anticipatory guidance about the normal "baby blues," outlines coping strategies, and encourages rest and support from family. Written materials and referral to a postpartum support group are provided.

This case illustrates the integration of **assessment, management, and education**, demonstrating how timely intervention prevents complications and reinforces self-care behaviors. The nurse's holistic approach supports both physiologic stability and emotional resilience.

Maternal postpartum nursing demands an equilibrium of clinical precision and empathy. Continuous monitoring of uterine tone, bleeding, and vital signs protects against immediate threats, while structured education prepares patients for independent care. Emotional awareness and family involvement elevate the quality of recovery, aligning with the broader goals of patient-centered nursing.

According to the provided material, the postpartum period is both a time of vulnerability and opportunity. Through anticipatory guidance, early recognition of complications, and compassionate communication, the nurse facilitates recovery that is not merely physical but deeply transformative.

Chapter 3 — Newborn Assessment and Management

The newborn period is characterized by rapid physiologic adaptation to extrauterine life. Nursing assessment focuses on recognizing normal transition processes and identifying deviations that require intervention. According to the provided material, the nurse's role encompasses comprehensive observation, evidence-based management, and ongoing parent education. Early recognition of subtle signs can prevent deterioration, emphasizing the critical nature of skilled assessment in the immediate postnatal period.

Physiologic Transition and Immediate Care

Upon birth, the newborn undergoes significant cardiovascular, respiratory, and thermoregulatory changes. Closure of the foramen ovale and ductus arteriosus redirects circulation, while pulmonary expansion facilitates oxygenation. Nurses ensure airway patency, stimulate breathing if necessary, and maintain warmth through skin-to-skin contact or radiant heat sources.

A **systematic initial assessment** includes evaluation of heart rate, respiratory effort, color, tone, and reflex irritability—elements of the Apgar score. This rapid appraisal determines the need for resuscitation or supportive measures. According to the provided material, most newborns transition effectively with minimal intervention; however, those who experience perinatal distress may require oxygen supplementation or bag-mask ventilation.

Thermoregulation remains a key priority. Heat loss occurs via evaporation, conduction, convection, and radiation. The nurse minimizes loss by drying the infant promptly, using warm linens, and maintaining environmental temperature. Hypothermia increases metabolic demands and may precipitate hypoglycemia, acidosis, and respiratory distress. Continuous monitoring ensures stability throughout the early adaptation period.

Comprehensive Newborn Assessment

The head-to-toe assessment provides a baseline for ongoing evaluation. Each observation contributes to understanding the newborn's physiologic status and adaptation.

- **Skin:** Color should be pink with possible transient acrocyanosis. Observe for jaundice, petechiae, or bruising. Vernix and lanugo indicate gestational maturity.
- **Head and Neck:** Assess fontanels for size and tension. A bulging fontanel may indicate increased intracranial pressure, while a sunken one suggests dehydration. Note molding, caput succedaneum, or cephalohematoma.
- **Eyes, Ears, and Mouth:** Confirm symmetry and patency. Epstein's pearls and milia are benign findings. Inspect for cleft lip or palate and ensure suck reflex integrity.
- **Cardiopulmonary:** Auscultate for murmurs, rate, and rhythm. Transient murmurs are common but should be reevaluated if persistent. Observe for nasal flaring, retractions, or grunting.
- **Abdomen and Umbilicus:** Soft and rounded; bowel sounds should be present within the first hour. Verify a three-vessel cord and monitor for drainage or redness.

- **Genitalia and Anus:** Confirm patency; note swelling due to maternal hormones.
- **Musculoskeletal:** Examine extremities for symmetry, tone, and range of motion. Check for hip instability using Ortolani or Barlow maneuvers.
- **Neurologic:** Reflexes such as Moro, rooting, and grasp demonstrate neurologic integrity.

Vital signs—temperature, heart rate, and respiratory rate—are recorded regularly, with glucose and bilirubin monitoring performed per policy. Nursing assessment emphasizes trend recognition rather than isolated readings, ensuring timely intervention.

Nursing Management and Family Education

Nursing management of the healthy newborn prioritizes stabilization, prevention of complications, and parent involvement. The nurse supports **bonding and attachment** through early contact, encouraging skin-to-skin care and rooming-in. According to the provided material, these practices promote thermoregulation, stabilize heart rate, and enhance breastfeeding success.

Feeding management is tailored to the newborn's needs. For breastfeeding infants, correct latch and frequent feeding every 2–3 hours maintain milk supply and glucose stability. Formula-fed infants require education on safe preparation, feeding intervals, and hygiene.

Monitoring for **elimination patterns** offers additional insight into hydration and renal function. The newborn should void within the first 24 hours and pass meconium shortly after birth. Delays may indicate anatomic or metabolic issues requiring evaluation.

Immunization and prophylactic care—administration of vitamin K and ophthalmic antibiotic—form part of standard practice. Screening tests, including metabolic panels and hearing evaluation, are completed before discharge. Nurses ensure parents understand the purpose of each procedure and provide reassurance throughout.

Discharge teaching encompasses **safe sleep**, cord care, temperature regulation, and recognition of distress signs such as poor feeding or persistent cyanosis. Encouraging open dialogue empowers families to respond promptly to concerns and fosters confidence in newborn care.

Thermoregulation and Metabolic Stability

Maintaining a stable body temperature is vital to neonatal survival and adaptation. The newborn's large surface area relative to weight and immature thermoregulatory mechanisms increase susceptibility to heat loss. According to the provided material, neutral thermal environment (NTE) maintenance is a core nursing responsibility, ensuring oxygen and glucose consumption remain minimal.

Four mechanisms of heat loss—**evaporation, conduction, convection, and radiation**—require active prevention strategies. Nurses immediately dry the infant after birth, remove damp linens, and use warmed surfaces. In the nursery, double wrapping or use of an incubator maintains consistent temperature. Regular monitoring of axillary temperature ensures early detection of deviations.

Cold stress results in peripheral vasoconstriction, hypoxemia, and metabolic acidosis as brown fat stores are metabolized for heat. Clinical signs include mottled skin, lethargy, and respiratory distress. Intervention involves rewarming gradually using skin-to-skin contact or servo-controlled devices. Conversely, **hyperthermia** may occur from environmental overheating or infection, presenting as flushed skin and tachypnea. Prompt cooling and investigation of underlying causes are essential.

Thermoregulatory stability supports metabolic balance. When temperature is controlled, glucose utilization remains efficient, preventing hypoglycemia—a condition often seen in preterm, small-for-gestational-age, or diabetic mothers' infants. Early feeding, whether breast or formula, stabilizes glucose levels and energy availability.

Feeding and Nutritional Management

Successful nutrition underpins growth, immunity, and neurodevelopment. The nurse's role includes assessing readiness for feeding, ensuring effective latch or bottle technique, and monitoring intake.

For breastfeeding infants, the first feeding should occur within the first hour after birth. Frequent feedings (8–12 per 24 hours) stimulate milk production and help regulate bilirubin levels through enhanced excretion. According to the provided material, effective latch indicators include rhythmic suck-swallow patterns and audible swallowing. The nurse assists with positioning and evaluates nipple comfort to prevent trauma.

Formula-fed infants require education on correct reconstitution and storage. Parents should be advised never to prop bottles and to discard unused formula after feeding. Measuring intake and output ensures adequate hydration.

Monitoring for **feeding difficulties**—such as poor suck, excessive sleepiness, or regurgitation—is essential. These may signal underlying metabolic or neurologic issues. The nurse promotes calm, low-stimulus feeding environments and supports paced feeding for preterm infants to prevent aspiration.

Elimination patterns provide indirect nutritional evidence. The newborn should produce at least one wet diaper per day of life for the first five days, progressing to six or more daily thereafter. Stool transitions from meconium to transitional and then to soft yellow by the end of the first week. Deviations, such as delayed stooling or persistent dark meconium, require evaluation.

Normal Patterns of Adaptation and Parental Teaching

Beyond physiologic stability, the nurse evaluates behavioral adaptation—sleep-wake cycles, reflex responsiveness, and bonding behaviors. The **quiet alert state** is optimal for interaction and feeding, while sleep phases support neurologic recovery. Educating parents about these states fosters understanding of newborn cues and promotes responsive caregiving.

Newborns display characteristic reflexes, including rooting, Moro, palmar grasp, and stepping, which indicate neurologic integrity. The nurse demonstrates these to parents, emphasizing their transient nature and developmental purpose.

Parental education remains integral to newborn management. Topics include:

- **Temperature regulation:** Dressing the infant in one more layer than adults wear, avoiding overheating.
- **Feeding cues:** Recognizing hunger signals—hand-to-mouth movement, rooting, and restlessness.
- **Sleep safety:** Always placing the infant supine on a firm surface free of soft objects.
- **Hygiene:** Gentle cord care, delayed bathing until thermal stability, and monitoring for redness or drainage.
- **Follow-up care:** Scheduling pediatric visits, newborn screening completion, and vaccination reminders.

By emphasizing understanding rather than rote compliance, nurses help families develop confidence and autonomy. According to the provided material, early mastery of newborn care tasks strengthens attachment and reduces anxiety, promoting positive long-term outcomes.

Screening and Ongoing Evaluation

Screening ensures early identification of disorders that might otherwise go undetected. According to the provided material, standard neonatal screenings include **metabolic, endocrine, hematologic, and auditory** assessments. Early detection allows for timely interventions that can prevent severe complications.

The **metabolic screen**, typically performed within 24–48 hours, detects disorders such as phenylketonuria, hypothyroidism, and galactosemia. **Hearing screening** identifies conductive or sensorineural loss, promoting early intervention and language development. **Critical congenital heart disease screening** using pulse oximetry assesses for oxygen desaturation and right-to-left shunting. Abnormal findings warrant immediate referral for further evaluation.

During hospitalization, nurses continue **daily assessment** for jaundice, feeding tolerance, and elimination patterns. The **transcutaneous bilirubin test** helps identify hyperbilirubinemia before it becomes clinically evident. Parental teaching emphasizes early detection of yellowing skin, poor feeding, or lethargy, which require medical attention.

By maintaining vigilant observation and encouraging parental participation, nurses ensure a seamless transition from hospital to home. The holistic management of the newborn concludes with discharge readiness and reinforcement of follow-up care.

Newborn nursing care integrates physiologic monitoring, environmental regulation, and comprehensive family education. According to the provided material, each intervention—from thermoregulation to feeding and bonding—serves to reinforce the newborn's adaptation to life outside the womb. Successful care depends on attention to detail, early recognition of deviations, and partnership with parents as primary caregivers.

Through compassionate instruction and evidence-informed practice, the nurse becomes both protector and educator, ensuring that each infant begins life within a safe and supportive environment.

Download Audio file and flashcards

Chapter 4 — Maternal Postpartum Complications

The postpartum period poses potential risks that, if undetected, can rapidly progress to life-threatening emergencies. Complications may arise from hemorrhage, infection, thromboembolism, hypertension, or psychological distress. According to the provided material, nurses play a pivotal role in early recognition, prompt intervention, and emotional support. Postpartum complication management requires an analytical blend of assessment skills and clinical reasoning grounded in pathophysiologic understanding.

Postpartum Hemorrhage (PPH)

PPH remains one of the leading causes of maternal morbidity and mortality worldwide. Defined as blood loss exceeding 500 mL after vaginal birth or 1000 mL after cesarean, it is often underrecognized until significant hypovolemia develops. **Uterine atony** is the most common etiology, characterized by a soft, poorly contracted uterus.

Nursing priorities include fundal assessment, evaluation of lochia amount, and observation for signs of hypovolemia such as tachycardia or pallor. Interventions begin with fundal massage, bladder emptying, and administration of uterotonic agents such as oxytocin or misoprostol as prescribed. If bleeding persists, escalation for provider evaluation is essential to identify lacerations, retained tissue, or coagulopathies.

According to the provided material, fluid resuscitation, oxygen therapy, and preparation for blood transfusion may be required. Continuous patient monitoring and emotional reassurance mitigate fear and anxiety during the event. Nurses also reinforce teaching regarding early warning signs after discharge, such as heavy bleeding or dizziness, prompting immediate medical attention.

Infection and Thromboembolic Complications

Postpartum infection may involve the uterus (endometritis), perineum, incision sites, or urinary tract. Risk factors include prolonged labor, multiple vaginal exams, and cesarean birth. Clinical manifestations include fever, uterine tenderness, and foul-smelling lochia. Nursing care emphasizes **hand hygiene, early ambulation, perineal care**, and adherence to antibiotic therapy as ordered.

Thromboembolic disorders, including deep vein thrombosis (DVT) and pulmonary embolism (PE), are linked to venous stasis and hypercoagulability. The nurse assesses for calf pain, swelling, warmth, or redness. Preventive measures include early mobilization, leg exercises, and use of compression devices. When diagnosed, management may involve anticoagulation under close monitoring.

Hypertensive disorders may persist postpartum. Eclampsia can occur even after delivery, with continued risk for seizures and stroke. Nurses monitor for headache, visual changes, or epigastric pain and ensure administration of antihypertensives or magnesium sulfate when prescribed.

The physical complications of the postpartum period often coincide with emotional vulnerability. The nurse's presence as a consistent and compassionate caregiver fosters trust, encouraging patients to report symptoms early. Holistic nursing practice acknowledges that recovery extends beyond the physical dimension, encompassing emotional and psychological health.

Psychological and Mood Disorders

The emotional well-being of a mother following childbirth is as vital as her physical recovery. The postpartum period may reveal a spectrum of psychological responses ranging from mild "baby blues" to severe psychiatric illness. According to the provided material, early identification and sensitive intervention are crucial components of nursing care.

The **postpartum blues**, experienced by nearly half of new mothers, typically manifest as mood swings, tearfulness, and fatigue beginning within the first week after delivery. These symptoms are transient, resolving within two weeks with rest, reassurance, and social support. However, **postpartum depression (PPD)** is more persistent, characterized by feelings of sadness, hopelessness, and loss of interest in activities or the infant. PPD can interfere with bonding and maternal functioning if unaddressed.

The most severe form, **postpartum psychosis**, is a psychiatric emergency presenting with delusions, hallucinations, or disorganized thinking. It often emerges within the first month postpartum and may endanger both mother and infant. Immediate psychiatric referral and safety measures are required.

Nursing responsibilities include routine emotional screening, active listening, and education about normal mood fluctuations. Encouraging open dialogue destigmatizes mental health and fosters trust. Nurses provide resources such as counseling services, peer support, and follow-up with healthcare providers. Families are taught to recognize early warning signs and seek help promptly.

Infectious Complications and Sepsis

Postpartum infection may arise in the uterus, urinary tract, breast, or surgical incisions. **Endometritis**, a common infection of the uterine lining, typically develops within the first 10 days postpartum. Clinical indicators include fever, abdominal pain, uterine tenderness, and malodorous lochia. The nurse monitors vital signs, encourages ambulation, promotes hydration, and administers prescribed antibiotics.

Wound infection occurs at perineal or cesarean sites. Redness, swelling, drainage, or delayed healing require immediate evaluation. Strict aseptic technique during perineal care and dressing changes reduces risk. For **urinary tract infections**, burning and urgency may indicate bacterial contamination; increasing fluid intake and antibiotic adherence aid resolution.

Mastitis, an infection of breast tissue, presents with localized tenderness, erythema, and flu-like symptoms. Continued breastfeeding or pumping is encouraged unless contraindicated, preventing milk stasis. Analgesics and warm compresses provide relief alongside antimicrobial therapy.

Severe or untreated infection can lead to **postpartum sepsis**, marked by systemic inflammatory response and potential organ dysfunction. Nurses maintain high vigilance for signs of hypotension, tachycardia, and altered mental status. Prompt notification of the healthcare provider, blood cultures, and initiation of intravenous fluids and antibiotics are key steps. According to the provided material, maternal sepsis demands multidisciplinary coordination and critical care readiness.

Nursing Response and Prevention Strategies

Proactive surveillance is the cornerstone of complication prevention. Postpartum nurses apply systematic approaches such as the **"BUBBLE-HE" assessment framework** (Breasts, Uterus, Bladder,

Bowels, Lochia, Episiotomy/Incision, Homan's Sign, Emotional Status). This comprehensive evaluation supports early detection of abnormalities.

Patient teaching reinforces self-assessment after discharge. Mothers are instructed to monitor for heavy bleeding, foul-smelling discharge, persistent fever, calf pain, or shortness of breath. Clear written instructions and follow-up calls enhance safety during the transition home.

Interdisciplinary collaboration amplifies nursing impact. Working alongside physicians, lactation consultants, and mental health professionals ensures holistic management. Infection control practices—hand hygiene, glove use, and environmental cleanliness—remain essential safeguards.

Emotional reassurance underpins every intervention. Recognizing fear and anxiety as natural responses to complications, nurses employ empathetic communication, maintaining a calm, confident presence. The integration of education, emotional support, and rapid action exemplifies the nurse's dual role as both guardian and guide through the complexities of postpartum recovery.

Recurrent Hemorrhage and Late-Onset Bleeding

While most postpartum hemorrhage (PPH) events occur within 24 hours, **secondary or late-onset hemorrhage** may develop days or weeks later. According to the provided material, this often results from subinvolution of the uterus, retained placental fragments, or infection. Symptoms include prolonged lochia rubra, uterine tenderness, and excessive bleeding.

Nursing management emphasizes assessment accuracy and early escalation. Palpation may reveal a boggy or enlarged uterus. Interventions include uterotonic medication administration as prescribed, patient education on rest, and avoidance of overexertion. Should infection be suspected, cultures and antibiotics are initiated promptly.

Patient teaching focuses on self-monitoring and reporting excessive bleeding, foul odor, or pelvic pain. Nurses provide reassurance that most secondary hemorrhage responds well to treatment when addressed early. Documenting blood loss accurately and maintaining interdisciplinary communication support continuity of care.

Hypertensive Sequelae and Long-Term Follow-Up

Hypertensive disorders such as **preeclampsia and eclampsia** can extend into or emerge after the postpartum period. Persistent headache, visual disturbances, or right upper quadrant pain warrant urgent evaluation. **Eclampsia**, marked by seizure activity, requires airway management, oxygen therapy, and magnesium sulfate administration.

According to the provided material, postpartum hypertension may persist for weeks and requires continued monitoring. Nurses reinforce medication adherence and scheduling of follow-up appointments. Education about lifestyle modification—nutrition, rest, and stress reduction—supports long-term vascular health.

Emotional support is integral; the lingering anxiety after a hypertensive emergency can affect maternal confidence. Nurses validate fears while reinforcing that recovery is achievable through continued surveillance and medical partnership.

Case Integration Example

A 33-year-old woman, four days post-cesarean, presents with fever, malaise, and incisional tenderness. Assessment reveals erythema and purulent drainage. The nurse notifies the provider, obtains a wound culture, and initiates prescribed antibiotics. Pain management and emotional reassurance accompany wound care teaching.

Two weeks later, she reports headaches and blurred vision. Blood pressure is 160/100 mmHg, consistent with postpartum hypertension. The nurse provides education regarding medication adherence and signs of eclampsia, emphasizing follow-up and safety.

This case underscores the **continuity of postpartum vigilance**—recognition that complications may unfold beyond initial discharge. Nursing competence lies in sustained observation, patient teaching, and multidisciplinary coordination, ensuring comprehensive maternal safety.

Chapter 4 Summary

Maternal postpartum complications demand decisive action, empathy, and advocacy. The nurse's role transcends detection; it encompasses prevention, intervention, and education. According to the provided material, consistent monitoring and communication remain the strongest defenses against morbidity. When complications arise, prompt evidence-based response transforms potential crises into recoverable events.

Chapter 5 — Newborn Complications

Newborn complications encompass a wide range of physiologic and developmental disturbances requiring rapid recognition and specialized care. According to the provided material, early detection of subtle signs is essential to prevent deterioration. The nurse's role includes continuous assessment, stabilization, and coordination with the healthcare team to achieve optimal outcomes.

Complications may be congenital, metabolic, infectious, or acquired through birth processes. Although each condition presents uniquely, the underlying principle remains constant: **timely intervention guided by physiologic understanding**.

Initial priorities focus on maintaining airway, temperature, and glucose stability while addressing the underlying cause. Emotional support for parents is critical; clear, compassionate explanations reduce anxiety and foster trust.

Neonatal Transition and Risk for Complications

At birth, the newborn undergoes rapid physiologic transformation as pulmonary gas exchange replaces placental oxygenation. The **Core Curriculum for Maternal–Newborn Nursing** describes this transition as dependent on alveolar fluid clearance, surfactant function, and cardiovascular shunting closure. Delays or failures in these processes create the foundation for early neonatal complications.

Infants most at risk include those born preterm, delivered via cesarean without labor, exposed to maternal diabetes, or experiencing perinatal asphyxia. Immediate postnatal assessment of respiration, tone, and color guides stabilization efforts as emphasized in **PCEP Specialized Newborn Care**, where accurate interpretation of early distress prevents escalation to respiratory failure.

Transient Tachypnea of the Newborn (TTN)

TTN represents the mildest and most common form of respiratory distress in term or near-term infants. It results from **delayed clearance of fetal lung fluid**, leading to interstitial edema and mild hypoxemia.

Typical onset occurs within the first two hours after birth. The *Core Curriculum* outlines hallmark signs: tachypnea (>60 breaths per minute), mild retractions, and nasal flaring, often resolving within 24 to 72 hours. Chest radiography shows prominent pulmonary markings and fluid in the fissures.

According to **Comprehensive Neonatal Nursing Care**, management focuses on supportive therapy—maintaining thermoneutrality, oxygen supplementation as needed, and avoidance of oral feeding until the respiratory rate stabilizes. Antenatal corticosteroids and delayed elective cesarean scheduling reduce risk by promoting surfactant maturation and fluid absorption.

Respiratory Distress Syndrome (RDS)

Formerly known as hyaline membrane disease, **RDS** primarily affects premature infants due to **surfactant deficiency** and structural lung immaturity. The *Comprehensive Neonatal Nursing Care* text notes that without adequate surfactant, alveoli collapse with each exhalation, causing atelectasis, decreased lung compliance, and impaired oxygen exchange.

Clinical presentation develops within minutes to hours: tachypnea, grunting, nasal flaring, and cyanosis. Radiographic imaging shows a "ground-glass" appearance with air bronchograms.
According to **PCEP Specialized Newborn Care**, management includes continuous positive airway pressure (CPAP) or mechanical ventilation, along with **exogenous surfactant administration** via endotracheal tube. Temperature regulation and minimal handling are crucial to reduce oxygen consumption.

Nurses must continuously monitor oxygen saturation, blood gases, and temperature, titrating inspired oxygen to prevent retinopathy of prematurity. Collaborative coordination with respiratory therapy ensures safe ventilation strategies and early weaning as lung compliance improves.

Meconium Aspiration Syndrome (MAS)

MAS occurs when meconium-stained amniotic fluid is aspirated into the lungs before or during delivery, leading to **airway obstruction, chemical pneumonitis, and surfactant inactivation**. The *Core Curriculum* highlights that it most frequently affects term or post-term infants experiencing intrauterine stress or asphyxia.

Clinical signs include respiratory distress, coarse breath sounds, and green-stained secretions. Chest imaging may reveal patchy infiltrates and areas of hyperinflation due to air trapping.
PCEP guidance emphasizes that vigorous infants should not undergo routine airway suctioning, whereas depressed infants may require tracheal suctioning under direct visualization prior to positive-pressure ventilation.

Management involves oxygen therapy, mechanical ventilation if needed, and in severe cases, **inhaled nitric oxide** or extracorporeal membrane oxygenation (ECMO). Continuous nursing surveillance includes pulse oximetry, arterial blood gas evaluation, and prevention of secondary infection.

Apnea of Prematurity

Apnea is defined as a **cessation of breathing for ≥20 seconds or shorter pauses associated with bradycardia or desaturation**. It reflects immaturity of central respiratory control, commonly seen in infants less than 34 weeks' gestation.

According to *Comprehensive Neonatal Nursing Care*, three patterns exist:

- **Central apnea** (absence of respiratory effort),
- **Obstructive apnea** (airflow obstruction with effort),
- **Mixed apnea** (combination of both).

Thermal instability, infection, or metabolic imbalance may exacerbate episodes. Continuous cardiorespiratory monitoring is mandatory. **Caffeine citrate** serves as the primary pharmacologic stimulant, increasing respiratory drive and reducing recurrence.

Nurses are advised to document episode frequency, associated events, and response to interventions. Gentle tactile stimulation is often sufficient; persistent apnea warrants assisted ventilation. The PCEP framework stresses maintaining neutral thermal environment and minimizing environmental stress to support neurologic maturation.

Persistent Pulmonary Hypertension of the Newborn (PPHN)

PPHN is a severe condition in which the **normal postnatal drop in pulmonary vascular resistance fails to occur**, causing continued right-to-left shunting and hypoxemia. The *Core Curriculum* attributes this to factors such as meconium aspiration, asphyxia, or congenital diaphragmatic hernia.

Clinical indicators include profound cyanosis despite oxygen administration, tachypnea, and differential oxygen saturation between pre- and post-ductal sites. Diagnosis is confirmed by echocardiography demonstrating right-to-left shunting at the ductus arteriosus or foramen ovale.

Management strategies from *PCEP Specialized Newborn Care* include high-frequency ventilation, inhaled nitric oxide to promote vasodilation, and maintenance of optimal systemic blood pressure. In refractory cases, ECMO provides temporary cardiopulmonary support.

Nursing roles encompass hemodynamic monitoring, thermal regulation, and strict avoidance of stimuli that provoke hypoxia-induced vasoconstriction. Families require clear explanations of technology and prognosis to reduce anxiety during intensive care.

Neonatal Pneumonia and Sepsis-Related Respiratory Failure

Infectious causes, particularly **group B streptococcus and gram-negative bacilli**, can produce respiratory distress indistinguishable from RDS. The *Core Curriculum* identifies maternal risk factors—prolonged rupture of membranes, chorioamnionitis, and prematurity.

Early-onset pneumonia presents within 72 hours, often with temperature instability, apnea, and poor feeding. Laboratory findings include leukopenia or elevated C-reactive protein.
Empiric antibiotic therapy (commonly ampicillin and gentamicin) begins after cultures are obtained, followed by adjustment based on results. Supportive nursing care mirrors that for RDS, emphasizing infection control, hand hygiene, and minimal stimulation.

Integrative Considerations: Maternal Link to Neonatal Respiratory Risk

Maternal health conditions directly shape neonatal outcomes. Diabetes predisposes infants to surfactant deficiency and RDS; hypertensive disorders correlate with intrauterine growth restriction and PPHN; and prolonged labor increases infection risk.

The *Core Curriculum* underscores the nurse's dual focus—recognizing how maternal complications inform newborn assessment and teaching families early signs of distress once discharged.
According to the *Comprehensive Neonatal Nursing Care* text, collaborative rounds involving both maternal and neonatal nurses optimize continuity of care and prevent missed warning signs during transition from birth unit to nursery or home.

Progress Note: This batch completes pages 42–49, concluding Chapter V: *Newborn Complications.* Coverage now includes thermoregulation, metabolic and infectious disorders, neurologic and cardiovascular complications, and end-of-Chapter synthesis. Chapter V is now **100% complete**.

Thermoregulation and Cold Stress

Newborns, especially preterm infants, are prone to **rapid heat loss** due to high surface area-to-mass ratio, thin skin, and limited subcutaneous fat. The *Core Curriculum for Maternal–Newborn Nursing* outlines the four modes of heat loss—evaporation, convection, conduction, and radiation.

Cold stress triggers increased oxygen consumption and metabolism of brown adipose tissue, leading to hypoglycemia and acidosis. According to *PCEP Specialized Newborn Care*, prevention begins at delivery: warm room temperature, immediate drying, skin-to-skin contact, and prewarmed equipment.

Signs include mottling, acrocyanosis, and lethargy. Management focuses on gradual rewarming, glucose monitoring, and maintaining a thermoneutral environment using radiant warmers or incubators. Continuous temperature surveillance is vital for stable perfusion and energy conservation.

Hypoglycemia

Defined by plasma glucose **<40 mg/dL in term** or **<30 mg/dL in preterm** infants, hypoglycemia is a frequent transitional disorder. The *Comprehensive Neonatal Nursing Care* text identifies risk groups: infants of diabetic mothers, small or large for gestational age, preterm, and those experiencing perinatal stress.

Clinical features—jitteriness, apnea, hypotonia, poor feeding, or seizures—require prompt assessment. Bedside glucose testing verifies diagnosis. **Early feeding** is first-line therapy; symptomatic infants or those unable to feed receive IV dextrose bolus followed by continuous infusion.
Nurses document pre- and post-intervention glucose values and monitor for rebound hypoglycemia. Maternal education stresses feeding frequency and recognition of recurrence at home.

Hyperbilirubinemia

Physiologic jaundice appears in most term infants after 24 hours, but pathologic elevation—rising **>5 mg/dL per day** or exceeding **15 mg/dL**—requires intervention. The *Core Curriculum* explains bilirubin as a breakdown product of fetal hemoglobin cleared via hepatic conjugation. Immature glucuronyl transferase or hemolysis overwhelms this system.

Phototherapy remains the cornerstone of management, converting bilirubin into excretable isomers. According to *PCEP Specialized Newborn Care*, optimal exposure, eye protection, hydration, and temperature maintenance are essential.
Severe untreated cases risk **kernicterus**, characterized by lethargy, high-pitched cry, and arching. Nursing vigilance and parental teaching regarding sunlight exposure, hydration, and follow-up bilirubin checks ensure safety after discharge.

Neonatal Sepsis

Neonatal sepsis is classified as **early-onset (<72 hours)** or **late-onset (>72 hours)**. The *Core Curriculum* cites **group B streptococcus and E. coli** as primary pathogens. Early-onset infection results from vertical transmission; late-onset typically reflects environmental exposure.

Symptoms are subtle—temperature instability, apnea, poor feeding, or pallor. Laboratory studies include blood culture, CBC with differential, and CRP. Empiric antibiotic therapy begins immediately after sampling, usually combining ampicillin and gentamicin.

Nursing responsibilities include strict aseptic technique, monitoring for toxicity, ensuring thermal and cardiorespiratory stability, and supporting family bonding during isolation precautions.
The *Comprehensive Neonatal Nursing Care* text emphasizes education on hygiene, cord care, and infection prevention in home settings, as recurrent infection risk persists in preterm infants.

Neurologic Complications

Hypoxic-ischemic encephalopathy (HIE) arises from perinatal asphyxia, manifesting with altered tone, seizures, and poor feeding. According to *Comprehensive Neonatal Nursing Care*, early identification permits initiation of **therapeutic hypothermia**—controlled cooling to 33.5 °C for 72 hours—to minimize brain injury.
Nursing care includes sedation management, continuous EEG monitoring, and prevention of shivering or hypotension.

Intraventricular hemorrhage (IVH) is another major risk in preterm infants, caused by fragile germinal matrix vessels. Graded I–IV by severity, it can lead to hydrocephalus or developmental delay. Monitoring involves cranial ultrasound, head circumference, and neurobehavioral observation. Maintaining stable oxygenation and minimizing handling reduce risk.

Parental counseling regarding prognosis and early-intervention referrals are integral to holistic nursing practice.

Cardiovascular Disorders

Patent ductus arteriosus (PDA) occurs when fetal shunting persists, allowing blood flow from aorta to pulmonary artery. The *Core Curriculum* outlines characteristic findings—murmur, widened pulse pressure, and bounding pulses.
Therapy includes **indomethacin or ibuprofen** to induce closure, or surgical ligation if medical management fails.
Congenital heart disease may first present as cyanosis or poor feeding. Pulse oximetry screening before discharge is mandated to detect critical defects early. Nurses must coordinate diagnostic follow-up and ensure parental comprehension of warning signs.

Shock—whether hypovolemic, cardiogenic, or septic—represents the final common pathway of decompensation. *PCEP Specialized Newborn Care* stresses rapid recognition, volume restoration, and thermoregulation to prevent multiorgan injury.

Gastrointestinal and Renal Complications

Feeding intolerance, vomiting, or abdominal distention may signal **necrotizing enterocolitis (NEC)**—a life-threatening inflammatory bowel disease of preterm infants. The *Comprehensive Neonatal Nursing Care* reference identifies early indicators: gastric residuals, abdominal discoloration, and apnea. Immediate interventions include stopping enteral feeds, initiating gastric decompression, and broad-spectrum antibiotics. Nursing care involves abdominal girth measurement, output monitoring, and minimizing handling. Parental support is critical during NPO status and possible surgical consultation.

Renal complications include acute tubular necrosis following hypoxia or dehydration. Monitoring urine output (minimum 1 mL/kg/hr), daily weight, and electrolyte trends guides therapy. Fluid balance is precise to prevent overload or deficit.

Metabolic acidosis secondary to sepsis or hypoxia manifests as tachypnea and lethargy. Correction requires addressing underlying causes and restoring perfusion.

Hematologic and Immune Disorders

Anemia of prematurity results from decreased erythropoietin and frequent sampling. *Core Curriculum* recommends iron supplementation and transfusion when clinically indicated.
Polycythemia—hematocrit >65%—increases viscosity, impairing perfusion and causing hypoglycemia or jaundice. Partial exchange transfusion may be required.
Isoimmunization (Rh or ABO incompatibility) can result in hemolytic disease, anemia, and jaundice. Prevention through maternal Rh immunoglobulin remains a key public health intervention, while exchange transfusion and phototherapy treat affected infants.

Integumentary and Musculoskeletal Complications

Pressure injuries and skin breakdown arise from adhesive trauma and medical devices. The *Comprehensive Neonatal Nursing Care* text promotes silicone-based dressings and gentle cleansing. For preterm infants, incubator humidity above 70% preserves barrier integrity.
Fractures and brachial plexus injuries may occur during difficult delivery. Immobilization, pain control, and gentle range-of-motion exercises aid recovery. Nursing documentation must include functional assessment at each shift.

Iatrogenic and Medication-Related Complications

Errors in infusion rates, phototherapy exposure, or medication dosing represent preventable causes of neonatal morbidity. PCEP emphasizes double-check protocols, standardized concentrations, and meticulous line labeling.
Extravasation injury from IV infiltration is prevented by hourly site inspection. When infiltration occurs, stop the infusion immediately and notify the provider; cold or warm compresses may be used depending on the agent.

Nurses serve as final safety barriers—verifying dose, route, and timing while maintaining situational awareness in complex NICU environments.

Family-Centered Support During Complications

Illness in the newborn disrupts the anticipated bonding process. The *Comprehensive Neonatal Nursing Care* framework stresses **family-integrated care**, where parents participate in decision-making, skin-to-skin contact when possible, and care activities suited to their infant's stability.
Cultural sensitivity, open communication, and psychosocial support reduce anxiety and foster resilience. Education on home monitoring, infection prevention, and medication administration promotes confidence post-discharge.

Ethical and Legal Considerations

Complex neonatal cases raise ethical questions surrounding resuscitation limits, surgical intervention, and quality of life. The *Core Curriculum* advises that decisions adhere to institutional policies and informed parental consent, balancing beneficence with respect for family autonomy.
Documentation must clearly reflect discussions, interventions, and outcomes. In end-of-life care, nurses uphold dignity through comfort positioning, pain control, and bereavement support.

Integration of Neonatal and Maternal Health Perspectives

The interdependence of maternal and neonatal outcomes remains central to the RNC-MNN® competency model. Maternal conditions—hypertension, infection, diabetes—mirror neonatal complications in predictable patterns.
Integrated charting, joint rounds, and transitional discharge planning are recognized by the *PCEP* and *Core Curriculum* texts as best practices ensuring safety and continuity across care settings.

Chapter 6 – Practice Questions

Questions (1-100)

Q1. A pregnant woman with pre-existing type 1 diabetes presents for prenatal care. Which complication is she most at risk for?

A. Placenta previa
B. Shoulder dystocia
C. Preeclampsia
D. Oligohydramnios

Q2. A client labor exhibits late decelerations on fetal monitoring. What is the priority nursing action?

A. Reposition the client laterally
B. Discontinue IV fluids
C. Prepare for immediate delivery
D. Apply fundal pressure

Q3. A woman at 34 weeks' gestation reports severe epigastric pain and blurred vision. Which is assessment finding supports the suspected diagnosis?

A. Proteinuria + severe hypertension
B. Low platelets and anemia
C. Painless vaginal bleeding
D. Premature rupture of membranes

Q4. A laboring patient develops uterine tachysystole after oxytocin infusion. What should the nurse do first?

A. Stop oxytocin infusion
B. Increase IV rate
C. Notify provider only
D. Administer uterotonic drug

Q5. A primigravida with placenta previa begins bleeding painlessly at 32 weeks. What is the initial nursing priority?

A. Perform vaginal exam
B. Assess fetal heart rate
C. Start oxytocin infusion
D. Administer tocolytics

Q6. A patient in the second stage of labor shows shoulder dystocia. Which maneuver is most appropriate?

A. McRoberts maneuver
B. Fundal pressure
C. Rapid vacuum extraction
D. Cesarean conversion

Q7. Which condition most increases risk for placental abruption?

A. Chronic hypertension
B. Gestational diabetes
C. Polyhydramnios
D. Multiple gestation

Q8. Which laboratory result suggests HELLP syndrome?

A. Elevated AST/ALT, low platelets, hemolysis
B. Low bilirubin only
C. Elevated BUN/creatinine alone
D. Increased WBC without anemia

Q9. A patient with preterm labor receives magnesium sulfate. Which assessment requires immediate attention?
A. Urinary output 40 mL/h
B. Warm flushing sensation
C. Mild nausea
D. Reflex score 0 and respirations 10/min
Q10. A laboring woman's membranes rupture and fetal heart rate drops suddenly. The nurse notes a palpable cord. Which action is first?
A. Relieve pressure on cord with hand
B. Prepare for tocolytic therapy
C. Document the finding and notify provider
D. Administer oxygen via nasal cannula
Q11. A laboring client with fever, tachycardia, and uterine tenderness is diagnosed with chorioamnionitis. What is the priority nursing action?
A. Obtain blood cultures and start antibiotics
B. Begin oxytocin induction
C. Administer tocolytics
D. Perform fundal massage
Q12. A 39-week gravida with ruptured membranes has a fetus in breech position. What complication is the nurse most concerned about?
A. Prolapsed umbilical cord
B. Placenta previa
C. Uterine rupture
D. Shoulder dystocia
Q13. A woman with preterm premature rupture of membranes (PPROM) at 30 weeks shows no infection. Which intervention is expected?
A. Discontinue IV fluids
B. Immediate induction of labor
C. Vaginal exam every 2 hours
D. Administer corticosteroids and observe
Q14. During delivery, meconium-stained amniotic fluid is noted. What should the nurse prepare for?
A. Neonatal airway suctioning and possible intubation
B. Immediate fundal massage
C. Maternal antibiotic therapy
D. Manual placental removal
Q15. A mother with Rh-negative blood delivers an Rh-positive infant. What nursing action prevents future hemolytic disease?
A. Administer Rho(D) immune globulin within 72 hours
B. Begin phototherapy immediately
C. Withhold breastfeeding for 24 hours
D. Give magnesium sulfate
Q16. A woman in labor develops sudden chest pain, dyspnea, and cyanosis after rupture of membranes. What is suspected?
A. Amniotic fluid embolism
B. Pulmonary infection
C. Placenta previa
D. Pulmonary edema from oxytocin

Q17. After vacuum-assisted delivery, a newborn shows poor tone and pallor. Which immediate nursing action is indicated?
A. Administer IV fluids
B. Stimulate and observe for 1 minute
C. Initiate positive-pressure ventilation
D. Obtain cord blood gases first
Q18. Which finding in a pregnant woman with hyperemesis gravidarum requires urgent attention?
A. Ketones in urine and dehydration
B. Mild nausea after breakfast
C. Small weight loss in first trimester
D. Heartburn after meals
Q19. A multipara presents with painful, dark vaginal bleeding and a rigid abdomen. Which complication is suspected?
A. Placental abruption
B. Placenta previa
C. Uterine rupture
D. Cervical insufficiency
Q20. A nurse caring for a woman with intrauterine growth restriction (IUGR) anticipates which fetal complication after birth?
A. Hypoglycemia
B. Polycythemia
C. Hypothermia
D. All of the above
Q21. A client at 28 weeks' gestation presents with BP 150/100 mm Hg and mild edema. Which finding differentiates chronic hypertension from gestational hypertension?
A. Onset before 20 weeks' gestation
B. Presence of proteinuria
C. Seizure activity
D. Headache after delivery
Q22. During a prenatal visit, a nurse educates a client with HIV. Which statement shows correct understanding?
A. "I'll take antiretroviral therapy throughout pregnancy."
B. "I'll avoid any medications to protect my baby."
C. "I should deliver vaginally to avoid anesthesia."
D. "I should stop breastfeeding for 2 months."
Q23. A woman with gestational diabetes has fasting glucose > 110 mg/dL despite diet. What is the next step?
A. Initiate insulin therapy
B. Repeat glucose tolerance test
C. Begin oral hypoglycemics
D. Restrict carbohydrates severely
Q24. A client in active labor shows fetal heart rate 90 bpm with recurrent variable decelerations. Which intervention should the nurse try first?
A. Administer magnesium sulfate
B. Start oxytocin infusion
C. Prepare for forceps delivery
D. Reposition to left lateral

Q25. A patient with ruptured membranes shows foul odor and fetal tachycardia. What complication should the nurse suspect?
A. Chorioamnionitis
B. Placental abruption
C. Amniotic fluid embolism
D. Uterine rupture
Q26. Which maternal condition increases risk for polyhydramnios?
A. Diabetes mellitus
B. Chronic hypertension
C. Placental insufficiency
D. Oliguria
Q27. A client in labor suddenly reports intense abdominal pain with cessation of contractions. Fetal heart tones are absent. Which emergency is likely?
A. Uterine rupture
B. Placental abruption
C. Cord prolapse
D. Shoulder dystocia
Q28. Which maternal infection requires cesarean delivery if active at labor onset?
A. Cytomegalovirus
B. Human papillomavirus
C. Hepatitis B
D. Genital herpes simplex
Q29. A nurse notes prolonged decelerations unresponsive to repositioning and oxygen. Which intervention is next?
A. Stop oxytocin and increase IV fluids
B. Continue current measures
C. Apply fundal pressure
D. Perform vaginal exam for descent
Q30. A patient with placenta accreta after prior cesarean experiences postpartum hemorrhage. Which treatment is most definitive?
A. Hysterectomy
B. High-dose oxytocin
C. Uterine massage
D. Manual placental removal
Q31. Which maternal condition increases risk for fetal neural-tube defects?
A. Folic-acid deficiency
B. Vitamin D toxicity
C. Iron overload
D. Zinc deficiency
Q32. A postpartum nurse suspects retained placental fragments. Which finding supports this?
A. Bradycardia and hypertension
B. Firm fundus with no lochia
C. Boggy uterus with continued bleeding
D. Elevated temperature 39 °C
Q33. Which fetal heart pattern indicates cord compression?
A. Variable decelerations
B. Early decelerations
C. Late decelerations

D. Sinusoidal pattern

Q34. A 17-year-old primigravida smokes one pack daily. Which fetal complication is most likely?

A. Intrauterine growth restriction
B. Polyhydramnios
C. Macrosomia
D. Neural-tube defect

Q35. A client in active labor experiences severe back pain with an occiput-posterior fetus. Which nursing intervention helps relieve discomfort?

A. Apply firm sacral counterpressure
B. Place client supine with knees flexed
C. Increase oxytocin infusion
D. Encourage breath-holding during contractions

Q36. A nurse prepares betamethasone for a 29-week client. What outcome indicates success?

A. Uterine relaxation
B. Improved fetal lung maturity
C. Reduced maternal BP
D. Increased amniotic fluid volume

Q37. Which sign differentiates placenta previa from abruption?

A. Painless bright-red bleeding
B. Rigid, tender uterus
C. Fetal distress
D. Abdominal pain

Q38. After delivery of a macrosomic infant, the nurse notes maternal hypotension and firm uterus. What complication is suspected?

A. Concealed internal bleeding (laceration)
B. Uterine atony
C. Placenta accreta
D. Retained membranes

Q39. A patient with multiple gestation presents in preterm labor. Which medication helps protect fetal neurodevelopment?

A. Magnesium sulfate
B. Terbutaline
C. Oxytocin
D. Indomethacin

Q40. A nurse assists with delivery of a newborn with thick meconium. Which step should occur immediately after birth?

A. Deep suction for all cases
B. Routine oropharyngeal suction first
C. Assess breathing and tone before suctioning
D. Delay assessment until cord clamping

Q41. A woman with chronic hypertension develops proteinuria at 30 weeks. What condition has likely developed?

A. Superimposed preeclampsia
B. Eclampsia
C. Gestational hypertension
D. Chronic renal disease

Q42. A nurse reviews labs for a pregnant client: hemoglobin 9 g/dL, MCV 70 fL. What nutrient deficiency is suspected?

A. Iron
B. Vitamin B12
C. Folic acid
D. Vitamin D

Q43. A nurse monitors a woman with oligohydramnios. Which fetal finding is expected?
A. Cord compression with variable decelerations
B. Polycythemia
C. Macrosomia
D. Hydrocephalus

Q44. Which assessment finding suggests labor progression in a patient with epidural analgesia?
A. Lower extremity weakness
B. Rising back pain
C. Decreasing blood pressure
D. Increasing pelvic pressure

Q45. After prolonged rupture of membranes (> 18 hours), what is the newborn most at risk for?
A. Neonatal sepsis
B. Hyperbilirubinemia
C. Hypoglycemia
D. Polycythemia

Q46. A nurse notes tachysystole and late decelerations after oxytocin initiation. Which drug should the nurse anticipate?
A. Terbutaline
B. Methylergonovine
C. Carboprost
D. Misoprostol

Q47. A postpartum woman exhibits restlessness, petechiae, and dyspnea after massive hemorrhage. What complication is suspected?
A. Disseminated intravascular coagulation (DIC)
B. Pulmonary embolism
C. Anaphylaxis
D. Endometritis

Q48. Which fetal presentation is most likely to cause prolonged labor?
A. Occiput anterior
B. Vertex flexed
C. Occiput posterior
D. Breech frank

Q49. A client with severe preeclampsia receives magnesium sulfate. Which parameter requires continuous monitoring?
A. Respiratory rate and reflexes
B. Urinary ketones
C. Temperature
D. Glucose levels

Q50. Which maternal lab finding is normal in healthy pregnancy?
A. Mild physiologic anemia
B. Elevated creatinine > 1.2 mg/dL
C. Thrombocytopenia < 100,000/mm^3
D. Positive proteinuria

Q51. A nurse evaluates a patient with preterm labor receiving tocolytics. Which assessment requires immediate reporting?
A. Maternal heart rate > 120 bpm
B. Blood pressure 110/70 mm Hg
C. Warm flushing sensation
D. Tremors of hands
Q52. After delivery, the newborn is floppy and cyanotic with no respirations. What is the first nursing action?
A. Suction stomach contents first
B. Begin chest compressions immediately
C. Administer oxygen by mask only
D. Dry and stimulate the infant on a warm surface
Q53. A nurse educates a patient on risk factors for preterm birth. Which statement indicates understanding?
A. "Stopping smoking and treating infections can help prevent early labor."
B. "Eating more carbohydrates causes premature delivery."
C. "Preterm birth can't be prevented."
D. "Exercise should be completely avoided."
Q54. A nurse assesses a postpartum patient who reports perineal pain and a feeling of fullness. The nurse notes firm fundus and continuous oozing of bright red blood. What is the most likely cause?
A. Uterine atony
B. Vaginal hematoma
C. Retained placental fragments
D. Cervical laceration
Q55. Which maternal vital sign pattern best indicates early postpartum hemorrhage?
A. Bradycardia and hypertension
B. Tachycardia with slight blood pressure drop
C. Bradypnea and hypotension
D. Normal vital signs until severe bleeding occurs
Q56. A nurse instructs a new mother about uterine involution. Which statement demonstrates correct understanding?
A. "My uterus should be back in my pelvis by two weeks."
B. "The uterus returns to prepregnancy size in three days."
C. "Fundus will remain palpable for a month."
D. "Involution is complete after six months."
Q57. A postpartum woman reports nipple pain during breastfeeding. Cracked, bleeding nipples are observed. The most appropriate initial nursing action is to:
A. Apply lanolin after feeding
B. Encourage longer feeding times
C. Verify infant latch and positioning
D. Pump breast milk exclusively
Q58. Lochia serosa typically appears during which postpartum period?
A. Days 1–3
B. Days 4–10
C. Days 11–21
D. After 4 weeks
Q59. During discharge teaching, which instruction is most appropriate to prevent mastitis?
A. Limit breastfeeding to every 4–6 hours

B. Wear a tight-fitting supportive bra
C. Empty breasts completely at each feeding
D. Apply ice packs before each feeding

Q60. Which symptom warrants immediate evaluation for postpartum depression?
A. Fatigue that improves with rest
B. Tearfulness resolving within two weeks
C. Persistent feelings of worthlessness and guilt
D. Anxiety about infant safety relieved by reassurance

Q61. A nurse evaluates lochia alba in a woman at 3 weeks postpartum. Which description is correct?
A. Bright red with small clots
B. Yellow-white with little odor
C. Pinkish-brown with foul smell
D. Gray-green mucopurulent discharge

Q62. Which intervention best promotes uterine contraction and reduces hemorrhage risk after birth?
A. Encourage ambulation within 12 hours
B. Massage fundus until firm
C. Administer stool softeners
D. Maintain lithotomy position

Q63. A nurse provides perineal care to a woman with an episiotomy. Which action is correct?
A. Apply ice for 24 hours, then warm sitz baths
B. Use heat immediately to reduce swelling
C. Avoid cleansing after urination
D. Delay sitz baths for one week

Q64. A postpartum patient experiences chills and fever 38.5 °C on day 3. The uterus is tender, lochia foul-smelling. What should the nurse suspect?
A. Mastitis
B. Endometritis
C. Cystitis
D. Wound infection

Q65. Teaching for cesarean section incision care includes which instruction?
A. Keep the dressing moist
B. Report redness or drainage
C. Remove steri-strips after 24 hours
D. Avoid showering for 10 days

Q66. Which finding indicates urinary retention after vaginal delivery?
A. Voiding 150 mL frequently
B. Urine output > 100 mL/hr
C. Burning with urination
D. Clear, odorless urine

Q67. A woman 4 days postpartum has firm, painful nodules in one breast with low-grade fever. Optimal action?
A. Stop breastfeeding until resolved
B. Continue feeding on affected side first
C. Apply cold compresses only
D. Begin prophylactic antibiotics

Q68. The nurse teaches contraception to a breastfeeding mother. Which method is most appropriate initially?
A. Combined oral contraceptive

B. Depo-Provera injection < 2 weeks postpartum
C. Progestin-only "mini-pill" after 6 weeks
D. Diaphragm within first 10 days

Q69. When assessing attachment, which maternal behavior indicates positive bonding?
A. Referring to infant as "it"
B. Touching infant with fingertips only
C. Smiling and talking to infant while feeding
D. Asking nurse to keep baby in nursery

Q70. Which dietary instruction aids iron recovery in a postpartum woman with mild anemia?
A. Drink milk with iron tablets
B. Take iron on empty stomach with juice
C. Avoid citrus when taking iron
D. Reduce protein intake

Q71. A woman 6 hours postpartum complains of dizziness when standing. Fundus is firm, vitals stable. Likely cause?
A. Postpartum hemorrhage
B. Orthostatic hypotension
C. Infection
D. Hypoglycemia

Q72. Teaching for Kegel exercises should include:
A. Perform while urinating each time
B. Contract pelvic muscles 10 times per set, 3 times daily
C. Avoid during first 6 weeks postpartum
D. Combine with abdominal crunches

Q73. A postpartum nurse observes moderate lochia rubra at 8 days postpartum. What is the best action?
A. Document as normal finding
B. Increase oral fluids
C. Notify provider of delayed involution
D. Encourage breastfeeding

Q74. A postpartum patient asks when she can resume sexual activity. Which nursing response is most accurate?
A. "You can resume as soon as you feel ready."
B. "After lochia stops and perineal healing occurs, usually about 4–6 weeks."
C. "Immediately after discharge."
D. "Wait three months."

Q75. Which finding requires urgent evaluation in a woman 2 weeks postpartum?
A. Mild breast engorgement
B. Yellow-white lochia
C. Passing large clots and bright-red bleeding
D. Light spotting after exertion

Q76. A nurse evaluates a postpartum woman complaining of calf pain and warmth. What is the priority nursing action?
A. Massage the affected area
B. Apply cold compress
C. Notify the healthcare provider
D. Encourage ambulation

Q77. Which intervention best supports a patient with postpartum urinary incontinence?

A. Restrict fluids to reduce leakage
B. Perform regular Kegel exercises
C. Use diuretics to control retention
D. Delay voiding to strengthen bladder

Q78. The nurse observes a mother crying and expressing fear she is a "bad mom" five days postpartum. Which intervention is most appropriate?
A. Notify psychiatry immediately
B. Reassure her that transient mood swings are common
C. Ignore the statement to avoid reinforcing negativity
D. Separate her from the infant temporarily

Q79. Which teaching should be emphasized for a postpartum patient taking iron supplements?
A. Take with milk to ease stomach upset
B. Avoid fiber to improve absorption
C. Expect dark stools as a normal effect
D. Discontinue if constipation occurs

Q80. A breastfeeding mother with cracked nipples asks about pain relief. The nurse's best advice is:
A. Apply alcohol wipes after feeds
B. Use expressed breast milk on nipples and air-dry
C. Stop breastfeeding for 48 hours
D. Wash nipples with soap each time

Q81. A nurse notes foul-smelling lochia and uterine tenderness in a woman 4 days postpartum. The nurse anticipates an order for:
A. Oral antifungal therapy
B. Broad-spectrum intravenous antibiotics
C. High-dose corticosteroids
D. Increased fluid intake only

Q82. The nurse teaches a postpartum woman about stool softeners. Which statement shows understanding?
A. "They prevent straining on my stitches."
B. "They'll stop all bowel movements for a week."
C. "I must stop breastfeeding while taking them."
D. "They may cause severe cramping."

Q83. Which behavior indicates effective maternal role adaptation?
A. Relies completely on staff for infant care
B. Expresses confidence in recognizing infant cues
C. Refuses to feed the baby without help
D. Describes newborn as difficult and unresponsive

Q84. A postpartum client with gestational diabetes asks about insulin needs after delivery. The nurse explains:
A. "You'll likely require more insulin postpartum."
B. "Your insulin requirement usually decreases after birth."
C. "Insulin is discontinued permanently."
D. "You must resume pre-pregnancy dosage immediately."

Q85. Which vital sign change is expected within the first 24 hours postpartum?
A. Fever > 39 °C
B. Bradycardia 50–60 bpm
C. Tachycardia > 120 bpm
D. Hypertension > 150/100 mm Hg

Q86. A woman reports severe perineal pain unrelieved by analgesics and minimal external swelling. The nurse suspects:
A. Vulvar hematoma
B. Normal episiotomy healing
C. Urinary retention
D. Endometritis
Q87. Which assessment finding signals hypovolemic shock in a postpartum patient?
A. Cool, clammy skin and rapid pulse
B. Flushed, warm skin and bounding pulse
C. Bradycardia with normal pressure
D. Slow respirations and warm extremities
Q88. A breastfeeding woman develops fever, localized breast redness, and malaise. Appropriate nursing guidance includes:
A. "Stop breastfeeding immediately."
B. "Continue feeding and begin prescribed antibiotics."
C. "Bind the breasts tightly."
D. "Use topical antifungal cream."
Q89. A postpartum woman complains of burning during urination and frequency. The nurse should suspect:
A. Normal postpartum diuresis
B. Cystitis
C. Uterine infection
D. Vaginal laceration
Q90. A nurse instructs on postpartum exercises. Which activity is safe within the first day after vaginal birth?
A. Leg and ankle movements while lying in bed
B. Sit-ups to strengthen abdomen
C. Jogging short distances
D. Lifting heavy objects
Q91. Which statement from a breastfeeding mother with adequate milk production reflects correct understanding of nutrition?
A. "I need 500 extra calories per day while nursing."
B. "I should restrict fluids to prevent engorgement."
C. "I'll return to my pre-pregnancy diet immediately."
D. "I should avoid calcium-rich foods."
Q92. On postpartum day 7, a patient experiences irritability, insomnia, and fatigue. Which evaluation is most important?
A. Advise bedrest for a week
B. Increase caffeine intake
C. Discontinue breastfeeding
D. Assess for postpartum depression onset
Q93. A nurse assesses a postpartum woman's fundus two hours after delivery. It is midline, firm, and at the level of the umbilicus. What action is indicated?
A. Document as normal finding
B. Massage until soft
C. Notify provider immediately
D. Increase IV fluids

Q94. The nurse provides discharge instructions to a woman 2 days postpartum. Which statement indicates correct understanding of perineal hygiene?
A. "I will clean front to back after using the toilet."
B. "I can use scented wipes to keep the area fresh."
C. "I'll skip cleansing if there is no bleeding."
D. "I should use hot compresses daily."
Q95. A nurse notes a saturated perineal pad within 15 minutes after delivery. What is the nurse's priority action?
A. Document as normal postpartum flow
B. Assess uterine tone and massage if boggy
C. Encourage the mother to rest
D. Administer an antipyretic
Q96. Which finding is considered normal when assessing a postpartum patient's breasts on day 3?
A. Soft and non-tender
B. Firm, warm, and tender to touch
C. Cold and pale
D. Red streaking and systemic fever
Q97. The nurse observes a postpartum woman sitting quietly, focusing on her newborn. This behavior best represents which maternal phase?
A. Taking-hold
B. Taking-in
C. Letting-go
D. Restorative
Q98. A patient asks how to relieve engorgement while continuing breastfeeding. The nurse should recommend:
A. Skip feedings to reduce supply
B. Limit fluid intake
C. Bind breasts tightly between feeds
D. Apply warm compresses before nursing
Q99. Which patient statement indicates proper understanding of lochia progression?
A. "Lochia should stay bright red for at least two weeks."
B. "It's normal for flow to increase after activity."
C. "If it smells foul, it's nothing to worry about."
D. "Clots the size of lemons can happen anytime."
Q100. Which assessment finding at 12 hours postpartum requires immediate intervention?
A. Firm fundus midline
B. Fundus deviated to the right
C. Scant lochia rubra
D. Soft breasts with colostrum

Answer key and Explanation (1-100)

Q1. Answer: B
Explanation: Diabetic mothers often deliver macrosomic infants, increasing risk for shoulder dystocia during birth. Preeclampsia and oligohydramnios may occur but are less directly linked to diabetes. Placenta previa is unrelated to glycemic control. Early glucose management reduces fetal overgrowth and delivery trauma.
Q2. Answer: A

Explanation: Late decelerations indicate uteroplacental insufficiency; lateral repositioning improves oxygen flow. Immediate delivery follows persistent distress. Fundal pressure worsens fetal hypoxia. Maintaining fluids supports perfusion; discontinuation would decrease circulation.
SubChapter: 1.2 Intrapartum Risk Factors

Q3. Answer: A

Explanation: Proteinuria and hypertension define preeclampsia, consistent with epigastric pain from liver involvement. Thrombocytopenia appears in HELLP but not always early. Painless bleeding suggests placenta previa, and ruptured membranes reflect infection risk not vascular spasm.
SubChapter: 1.3 Complications of Pregnancy

Q4. Answer: A

Explanation: Excessive contractions decrease placental perfusion; stopping oxytocin immediately prevents fetal distress. Increasing IV rate or administering more uterotonics worsens tachysystole. The provider must be notified after the infusion is stopped to evaluate fetal status.
SubChapter: 1.2 Intrapartum Risk Factors

Q5. Answer: B

Explanation: Fetal assessment guides urgency of intervention in placenta previa. Vaginal exam is contraindicated because it can trigger profuse bleeding. Oxytocin or tocolytics are secondary to stabilizing mother and fetus first.
SubChapter: 1.3 Complications of Pregnancy

Q6. Answer: A

Explanation: McRoberts maneuver flexes the thighs to open the pelvic outlet, releasing the shoulder. Fundal pressure and vacuum increase fetal injury risk; cesarean follows failed maneuvers. Prompt team response reduces neonatal asphyxia.
SubChapter: 1.4 Complications of Birth and Transition

Q7. Answer: A

Explanation: Hypertension causes placental vessel damage, predisposing to abruption. Gestational diabetes and polyhydramnios increase uterine distension but not detachment. Multiple gestation may stretch the uterus but is less direct than vascular pathology.
SubChapter: 1.1 Antenatal Risk Factors

Q8. Answer: A

Explanation: HELLP stands for Hemolysis, Elevated Liver enzymes, Low Platelets. It is a severe preeclampsia variant requiring delivery. Isolated bilirubin or renal changes do not define HELLP, and infection may raise WBC but lacks hemolysis.
SubChapter: 1.3 Complications of Pregnancy

Q9. Answer: D

Explanation: Absent reflexes and respiratory depression indicate toxicity. Flushing and nausea are expected side effects; urinary output ≥ 30 mL/h is adequate for excretion. Calcium gluconate should be readily available as antidote.
SubChapter: 1.3 Complications of Pregnancy

Q10. Answer: A

Explanation: Manual relief of cord compression restores oxygenation until emergency delivery. Oxygen and notification follow immediately. Tocolytics may be considered later but not before relieving cord pressure.
SubChapter: 1.4 Complications of Birth and Transition

Q11. Answer: A

Explanation: Infection within the uterus threatens mother and fetus; cultures and antibiotics prevent sepsis. Induction may follow once infection control starts. Tocolytics worsen infection risk, and fundal massage addresses postpartum atony, not intrapartum infection.

SubChapter: 1.2 Intrapartum Risk Factors
Q12. Answer: A
Explanation: Breech with ruptured membranes allows cord descent before the presenting part, risking compression and fetal hypoxia. Placenta previa involves implantation site, uterine rupture stems from scar stress, and shoulder dystocia occurs with cephalic macrosomia.
SubChapter: 1.2 Intrapartum Risk Factors
Q13. Answer: D
Explanation: Corticosteroids promote fetal lung maturity while observation monitors infection onset. Induction risks prematurity; repeated exams raise infection; adequate hydration maintains uteroplacental flow. Expectant management balances maternal–fetal safety.
SubChapter: 1.3 Complications of Pregnancy
Q14. Answer: A
Explanation: Meconium aspiration threatens airway obstruction; resuscitation team prepares for suction or intubation. Fundal massage follows birth for tone; antibiotics target infection, not aspiration; placental removal is unrelated.
SubChapter: 1.4 Complications of Birth and Transition
Q15. Answer: A
Explanation: Rho(D) immune globulin prevents maternal antibody formation after fetal–maternal mixing. Phototherapy treats newborn jaundice, breastfeeding is unrelated, and magnesium sulfate is for preeclampsia seizure prevention. Timely prophylaxis ensures future fetal safety.
SubChapter: 1.1 Antenatal Risk Factors
Q16. Answer: A
Explanation: Sudden cardiovascular collapse after membrane rupture signals amniotic fluid embolism, an obstetric emergency needing resuscitation. Infection and pulmonary edema progress slower, while previa causes bleeding without respiratory failure. Rapid recognition saves lives.
SubChapter: 1.3 Complications of Pregnancy
Q17. Answer: C
Explanation: Depressed respirations and tone require ventilation per neonatal resuscitation guidelines. Observation delays oxygenation; IV fluids and gases follow stabilization. Prompt ventilation prevents hypoxic injury and supports transition to extrauterine life.
SubChapter: 1.4 Complications of Birth and Transition
Q18. Answer: A
Explanation: Ketonuria and dehydration indicate severe metabolic imbalance needing IV therapy. Mild nausea and heartburn are typical, and small weight loss is often benign. Persistent vomiting jeopardizes electrolyte and fetal growth status.
SubChapter: 1.1 Antenatal Risk Factors
Q19. Answer: A
Explanation: Painful bleeding with uterine rigidity defines placental abruption from premature separation. Previa bleeding is painless, rupture shows fetal parts and sudden pain after scar stress, and insufficiency occurs without pain in mid-pregnancy.
SubChapter: 1.3 Complications of Pregnancy
Q20. Answer: D
Explanation: IUGR infants have low glycogen stores, poor temperature regulation, and increased erythropoietin from hypoxia causing polycythemia. Recognizing these risks guides early monitoring, glucose support, and thermal management to prevent morbidity.
SubChapter: 1.1 Antenatal Risk Factors
Q21. Answer: A

Explanation: Hypertension present before 20 weeks indicates chronic hypertension. Gestational hypertension develops after 20 weeks without proteinuria. Seizures define eclampsia, and postpartum headache is nonspecific. Early identification guides appropriate monitoring.
SubChapter: 1.1 Antenatal Risk Factors

Q22. Answer: A

Explanation: Continuous antiretroviral therapy reduces vertical transmission dramatically. Withholding treatment endangers both. Vaginal birth and breastfeeding depend on viral load and national policy, but medication adherence remains cornerstone prevention.
SubChapter: 1.1 Antenatal Risk Factors

Q23. Answer: A

Explanation: Insulin is preferred for uncontrolled gestational diabetes when diet fails, maintaining tight glucose control for fetal safety. Oral agents cross placenta variably, severe restriction risks ketosis, and repeating tests delays management.
SubChapter: 1.1 Antenatal Risk Factors

Q24. Answer: D

Explanation: Variable decelerations suggest cord compression; lateral positioning relieves pressure. Oxytocin worsens stress, forceps are premature, and magnesium isn't indicated. Repositioning is quick and often effective.
SubChapter: 1.2 Intrapartum Risk Factors

Q25. Answer: A

Explanation: Foul amniotic odor and fetal tachycardia indicate intra-amniotic infection. Abruption involves pain and bleeding, embolism causes cardiovascular collapse, and rupture presents with sudden pain after scar stress. Prompt antibiotics are essential.
SubChapter: 1.2 Intrapartum Risk Factors

Q26. Answer: A

Explanation: Fetal hyperglycemia from diabetic mothers leads to osmotic diuresis and excess amniotic fluid. Hypertension and placental insufficiency more often cause oligohydramnios, and oliguria decreases—not increases—fluid. Monitoring prevents preterm labor.
SubChapter: 1.1 Antenatal Risk Factors

Q27. Answer: A

Explanation: Uterine rupture causes tearing pain, loss of tone, and fetal distress. Abruption shows ongoing contractions with bleeding; cord prolapse manifests with variable decelerations; shoulder dystocia occurs during delivery. Immediate surgery is vital.
SubChapter: 1.2 Intrapartum Risk Factors

Q28. Answer: D

Explanation: Active genital herpes lesions risk neonatal encephalitis; cesarean prevents exposure. HPV rarely transmits perinatally, and hepatitis B or CMV manage via post-exposure prophylaxis, not cesarean mandate.
SubChapter: 1.1 Antenatal Risk Factors

Q29. Answer: A

Explanation: Decreasing oxytocin and boosting fluids improve uteroplacental perfusion. Fundal pressure may worsen compression; repetitive exams delay response. Persistent decelerations require intrauterine resuscitation steps before operative delivery.
SubChapter: 1.2 Intrapartum Risk Factors

Q30. Answer: A

Explanation: Placenta accreta invades the uterine wall, preventing separation; hysterectomy controls life-threatening bleeding. Oxytocin and massage treat atony, not invasion. Manual removal risks catastrophic hemorrhage.

SubChapter: 1.3 Complications of Pregnancy

Q31. Answer: A

Explanation: Folic acid supports neural-tube closure; deficiency leads to spina bifida or anencephaly. Vitamin D, iron, and zinc imbalances affect other systems but not primary neural development. Early supplementation prevents defects.

SubChapter: 1.1 Antenatal Risk Factors

Q32. Answer: C

Explanation: Retained fragments prevent full uterine contraction, producing bogginess and bleeding. A firm fundus indicates atony correction; fever suggests infection. Prompt evacuation prevents hemorrhagic shock.

SubChapter: 1.3 Complications of Pregnancy

Q33. Answer: A

Explanation: Variable decelerations vary in timing and shape, reflecting cord compression. Early decels mirror contractions (head compression), late decels show hypoxia, sinusoidal patterns imply severe anemia. Recognizing variables guides prompt repositioning.

SubChapter: 1.2 Intrapartum Risk Factors

Q34. Answer: A

Explanation: Smoking causes vasoconstriction and hypoxia, restricting growth. Polyhydramnios and macrosomia stem from diabetes, while neural-tube defects relate to folate deficiency. Smoking cessation improves placental perfusion and fetal outcome.

SubChapter: 1.1 Antenatal Risk Factors

Q35. Answer: A

Explanation: Counterpressure relieves back pain from fetal occiput against sacrum. Supine position decreases perfusion; more oxytocin or breath-holding worsen distress. Non-pharmacologic measures aid maternal coping.

SubChapter: 1.2 Intrapartum Risk Factors

Q36. Answer: B

Explanation: Betamethasone accelerates surfactant production to reduce respiratory distress syndrome in preterm infants. It does not relax the uterus, affect BP, or change fluid levels. Corticosteroid timing is critical before delivery.

SubChapter: 1.3 Complications of Pregnancy

Q37. Answer: A

Explanation: Placenta previa causes painless, bright bleeding from lower-segment implantation. Abruption presents with painful, firm uterus and distress. Distinguishing them determines safe delivery planning and hemorrhage precautions.

SubChapter: 1.3 Complications of Pregnancy

Q38. Answer: A

Explanation: A firm uterus with ongoing bleeding indicates genital-tract laceration rather than atony. Accreta and retained membranes cause boggy uterus or delayed bleeding. Rapid inspection and repair prevent shock.

SubChapter: 1.4 Complications of Birth and Transition

Q39. Answer: A

Explanation: Magnesium sulfate provides fetal neuroprotection and seizure prophylaxis if preeclampsia coexists. Terbutaline and indomethacin are tocolytics; oxytocin induces contractions. Proper dosing minimizes respiratory depression.

SubChapter: 1.3 Complications of Pregnancy

Q40. Answer: C

Explanation: Current guidelines recommend assessing vigor first; suction only if poor tone or apnea. Routine deep suction can cause trauma. Rapid evaluation ensures proper airway management without unnecessary intervention.
SubChapter: 1.4 Complications of Birth and Transition
Q41. Answer: A
Explanation: Proteinuria emerging after mid-pregnancy in a hypertensive patient signals superimposed preeclampsia, requiring close monitoring. Eclampsia adds seizures, gestational hypertension lacks proteinuria, and chronic renal disease predates conception. Early identification prevents severe complications.
SubChapter: 1.1 Antenatal Risk Factors
Q42. Answer: A
Explanation: Microcytic anemia (low MCV) points to iron deficiency, common in pregnancy due to increased demand. Vitamin B12 and folate deficiencies cause macrocytosis, and vitamin D affects bone metabolism, not red-cell size. Supplementation restores oxygen-carrying capacity.
SubChapter: 1.1 Antenatal Risk Factors
Q43. Answer: A
Explanation: Low amniotic fluid limits cushioning, increasing cord compression and variable decelerations. Polycythemia and macrosomia relate to diabetes, hydrocephalus enlarges head size but not fluid volume. Close surveillance reduces hypoxia risk.
SubChapter: 1.1 Antenatal Risk Factors
Q44. Answer: D
Explanation: Epidural blocks pain perception; increasing pelvic pressure signals descent and impending birth. Back pain indicates early labor, hypotension is a side effect not progression, and leg weakness reflects motor block. Ongoing assessment ensures timely preparation.
SubChapter: 1.2 Intrapartum Risk Factors
Q45. Answer: A
Explanation: Extended membrane rupture invites ascending infection leading to neonatal sepsis. Jaundice, hypoglycemia, and polycythemia relate to metabolic or hypoxic causes, not direct infection risk. Prompt maternal antibiotics reduce transmission.
SubChapter: 1.4 Complications of Birth and Transition
Q46. Answer: A
Explanation: Terbutaline, a beta-agonist, relaxes uterine muscle to relieve tachysystole. Methylergonovine and carboprost increase tone and would worsen distress; misoprostol induces labor. Quick tocolysis protects fetal oxygenation.
SubChapter: 1.2 Intrapartum Risk Factors
Q47. Answer: A
Explanation: DIC follows major bleeding or abruption, manifesting with petechiae and respiratory distress from microthrombi. Pulmonary embolism causes sudden pain without bleeding signs; anaphylaxis has hypotension; endometritis shows fever. Rapid support and blood products are critical.
SubChapter: 1.3 Complications of Pregnancy
Q48. Answer: C
Explanation: Occiput posterior delays descent due to malalignment of the fetal head, prolonging labor and back pain. Vertex flexed and anterior positions promote efficient delivery; breech often requires cesarean but not prolonged labor once delivery starts.
SubChapter: 1.2 Intrapartum Risk Factors
Q49. Answer: A

Explanation: Magnesium depresses neuromuscular activity; respiratory rate < 12 or absent reflexes signal toxicity. Ketones, temperature, and glucose aren't directly affected. Calcium gluconate must be available for reversal. Frequent assessment prevents arrest.
SubChapter: 1.3 Complications of Pregnancy

Q50. Answer: A

Explanation: Increased plasma volume dilutes red cells causing physiologic anemia. Creatinine and proteinuria should decrease in normal pregnancy; thrombocytopenia suggests preeclampsia or HELLP. Recognizing normal shifts prevents unnecessary intervention.
SubChapter: 1.1 Antenatal Risk Factors

Q51. Answer: A

Explanation: Beta-agonist tocolytics may cause tachycardia; > 120 bpm signals excess stimulation. Flushing and tremors are expected; BP 110/70 is normal. Reporting allows dose adjustment and prevention of cardiac stress.
SubChapter: 1.3 Complications of Pregnancy

Q52. Answer: D

Explanation: Initial neonatal resuscitation focuses on warming and stimulation to trigger respiration. If ineffective after 30 seconds, positive-pressure ventilation follows. Immediate compressions or oxygen without assessment delays effective care.
SubChapter: 1.4 Complications of Birth and Transition

Q53. Answer: A

Explanation: Smoking and infection increase prostaglandin activity that triggers labor; eliminating these reduces risk. Diet composition and moderate exercise don't directly cause prematurity. Education empowers preventive self-care.
SubChapter: 1.1 Antenatal Risk Factors
Chapter 2

Q54. Answer: B

Explanation: A firm uterus with persistent bleeding suggests trauma rather than atony; a vaginal hematoma causes localized pain, pressure, and concealed bleeding. Option A – Atony causes boggy uterus. Option C – Retained fragments cause boggy tone. Option D – Lacerations show visible bright bleeding.
SubChapter: Maternal Assessment & Hemorrhage Recognition

Q55. Answer: B

Explanation: Tachycardia is an early compensatory response to blood loss, preceding hypotension. Option A – Bradycardia is atypical. Option C – Bradypnea appears in shock. Option D – Vital changes occur before late stage hemorrhage.
SubChapter: Hemodynamic Monitoring After Birth

Q56. Answer: A

Explanation: After birth, uterine fundus descends approximately 1 cm/day and becomes nonpalpable by two weeks. Option B – Too rapid. Option C – Too long. Option D – Extremely delayed.
SubChapter: Postpartum Physical Assessment

Q57. Answer: C

Explanation: Poor latch is the most common cause of nipple trauma; correcting positioning promotes healing and comfort. Option A – Adjunct therapy only. Option B – Worsens injury. Option D – Temporary if severe damage.
SubChapter: Lactation Support & Education

Q58. Answer: B

Explanation: Lochia serosa (pink or brown) follows lochia rubra and lasts approximately 4–10 days postpartum. Option A – Rubra stage. Option C – Alba stage. Option D – Abnormal persistence indicates infection.
SubChapter: Uterine Involution & Lochial Pattern

Q59. Answer: C

Explanation: Frequent, complete emptying prevents milk stasis and infection. Option A – Infrequent feeding promotes stasis. Option B – Constriction impedes flow. Option D – Ice decreases let-down reflex.
SubChapter: Breast Care & Infection Prevention

Q60. Answer: C

Explanation: Persistent guilt and worthlessness beyond 2 weeks signify major depression needing intervention. Option A – Normal fatigue. Option B – Typical "baby blues." Option D – Common early anxiety.
SubChapter: Psychologic Adaptation & Education

Q61. Answer: B

Explanation: Lochia alba is pale yellow-white, scant, and nearly odorless, marking final uterine healing. Option A – Early rubra stage. Option C – Suggests infection. Option D – Purulent, abnormal.
SubChapter: Lochial Assessment & Patient Education

Q62. Answer: B

Explanation: Fundal massage stimulates uterine tone and constricts blood vessels, reducing hemorrhage. Option A – Prevents thrombosis but not contraction. Option C – Unrelated. Option D – Not therapeutic.
SubChapter: Immediate Postpartum Hemorrhage Prevention

Q63. Answer: A

Explanation: Cold therapy minimizes swelling for 24 hours, followed by heat to enhance circulation and comfort. Option B – Increases edema early. Option C – Increases infection risk. Option D – Unnecessary delay.
SubChapter: Perineal Care & Comfort Measures

Q64. Answer: B

Explanation: Endometritis presents with uterine tenderness, foul lochia, and fever typically within 2–5 days. Option A – Breast localized. Option C – Urinary symptoms. Option D – Incision redness.
SubChapter: Postpartum Infection Recognition

Q65. Answer: B

Explanation: Redness or drainage indicates infection and must be reported promptly. Option A – Moisture encourages infection. Option C – Allow natural detachment. Option D – Gentle showering acceptable after 48 hours.
SubChapter: Cesarean Wound Care & Teaching

Q66. Answer: A

Explanation: Small, frequent voids suggest incomplete emptying due to bladder atony or edema. Option B – Normal output. Option C – Suggests infection. Option D – Normal appearance.
SubChapter: Elimination Assessment Post-Birth

Q67. Answer: B

Explanation: Breast emptying through continued feeding relieves blocked ducts; start on affected side. Option A – Aggravates stasis. Option C – May relieve pain but not obstruction. Option D – Not indicated unless infection develops.
SubChapter: Lactation Complication Management

Q68. Answer: C

Explanation: Progestin-only pills are safe for breastfeeding and initiated ≥ 6 weeks postpartum. Option A – Estrogen reduces milk. Option B – Too early for hormonal use. Option D – Pelvic support not restored.

SubChapter: Postpartum Contraceptive Counseling

Q69. Answer: C

Explanation: Eye contact, smiling, and verbal interaction reflect maternal-infant attachment. Option A – Detachment. Option B – Initial stage only. Option D – Avoidance behavior.

SubChapter: Parent–Infant Bonding Assessment

Q70. Answer: B

Explanation: Vitamin C enhances iron absorption; best taken on empty stomach with juice. Option A – Calcium inhibits absorption. Option C – Opposite advice. Option D – Protein supports healing.

SubChapter: Postpartum Nutrition Education

Q71. Answer: B

Explanation: Blood volume shifts and vasodilation cause transient orthostatic hypotension; rise slowly to prevent falls. Option A – Would show tachycardia. Option C – Fever absent. Option D – No glucose symptoms.

SubChapter: Safety & Physiologic Adaptation

Q72. Answer: B

Explanation: Kegels strengthen pelvic floor; ten contractions × three sets daily restore tone. Option A – Occasional testing only. Option C – May start once comfortable. Option D – Unrelated muscles.

SubChapter: Pelvic Rehabilitation Teaching

Q73. Answer: C

Explanation: Rubra persisting > 7 days suggests subinvolution or retained tissue; provider evaluation required. Option A – Not normal beyond week 1. Option B – No effect on bleeding. Option D – Helps contraction but needs assessment.

SubChapter: Assessment of Uterine Involution

Q74. Answer: B

Explanation: Resumption of intercourse is safe when perineal tissues have healed, lochia has ceased, and the cervix has closed—commonly between four and six weeks postpartum. Early activity increases infection and bleeding risk; waiting several months is unnecessary unless complications arise.

SubChapter: Postpartum Sexual Health Education

Q75. Answer: C

Explanation: Return of bright-red bleeding with clots after lochia has lightened suggests secondary hemorrhage or retained fragments, demanding immediate provider assessment. Minor spotting or engorgement is expected; lochia alba is normal transition. Prompt recognition prevents severe anemia or infection progression.

SubChapter: Abnormal Lochia & Hemorrhage Assessment

Q76. Answer: C

Explanation: Localized pain, heat, and swelling may indicate deep-vein thrombosis requiring urgent medical evaluation to prevent embolism. Massage or early ambulation could dislodge the clot. Prompt reporting ensures diagnostic confirmation and timely anticoagulant therapy.

SubChapter: Circulatory Assessment & Safety

Q77. Answer: B

Explanation: Kegel exercises restore pelvic floor muscle tone, improving bladder control without compromising hydration. Fluid restriction or delayed voiding increases infection and retention risk, while diuretics may worsen dehydration. Consistent exercise promotes long-term continence and patient confidence.

SubChapter: Pelvic Floor Rehabilitation

Q78. Answer: B

Explanation: "Baby blues" often occur within the first week due to hormonal shifts, fatigue, and stress. Supportive reassurance, rest, and help with newborn care usually resolve symptoms. Persistent sadness beyond two weeks signals depression and requires referral.
SubChapter: Psychologic Adaptation & Counseling
Q79. Answer: C
Explanation: Iron commonly darkens stools and may cause mild constipation; these are normal effects, not toxicity signs. Milk and antacids reduce absorption, while adequate fiber and fluids help prevent constipation, supporting continued therapy compliance and iron repletion.
SubChapter: Nutritional Management & Education
Q80. Answer: B
Explanation: Expressed milk contains natural antimicrobial and healing factors; air-drying soothes soreness. Alcohol and soap dry tissues and delay healing. Continuing frequent, correct-latch feeding prevents engorgement and maintains supply while tissues recover safely.
SubChapter: Breastfeeding Technique & Comfort
Q81. Answer: B
Explanation: These signs indicate endometritis, a uterine bacterial infection managed with broad-spectrum IV antibiotics and supportive care. Antifungals and steroids are inappropriate; hydration alone is insufficient. Early treatment prevents sepsis and fertility complications.
SubChapter: Postpartum Infection Management
Q82. Answer: A
Explanation: Stool softeners ease defecation, reducing pressure on perineal sutures and hemorrhoids. They do not halt bowel function, are safe during lactation, and rarely cause cramping. Preventing constipation supports healing and comfort during recovery.
SubChapter: Elimination Management & Patient Teaching
Q83. Answer: B
Explanation: Confidence in identifying and responding to infant needs reflects successful maternal adaptation. Dependence or negative perceptions suggest delayed adjustment. Positive feedback and education reinforce competence and strengthen mother-infant attachment during postpartum transition.
SubChapter: Parenting Role Transition
Q84. Answer: B
Explanation: After placental delivery, insulin-antagonistic hormones drop, reducing maternal insulin needs. Blood glucose monitoring guides adjustments. Permanent discontinuation or automatic resumption of old doses may cause hypo- or hyperglycemia; individualized management ensures metabolic stability.
SubChapter: Endocrine Adjustment & Education
Q85. Answer: B
Explanation: Transient bradycardia results from increased stroke volume after blood loss replacement and diuresis. Persistent tachycardia or fever indicates infection or hemorrhage, and hypertension warrants evaluation for preeclampsia. Understanding physiologic adaptation helps nurses differentiate normal from pathologic changes.
SubChapter: Vital Sign Monitoring Postpartum
Q86. Answer: A
Explanation: Deep, unrelenting perineal pain with little visible swelling indicates a vulvar or vaginal hematoma from vessel injury. Prompt recognition allows incision and evacuation. Routine healing pain responds to analgesics; urinary or uterine issues present differently.
SubChapter: Perineal Assessment & Trauma Care
Q87. Answer: A

Explanation: Pale, clammy skin and tachycardia indicate decreased perfusion from volume loss. Bounding pulse and warmth suggest opposite states. Immediate fluid resuscitation and uterotonic therapy prevent organ failure and mortality.
SubChapter: Emergency Hemorrhage Response
Q88. Answer: B
Explanation: Mastitis management involves continued milk removal, rest, and antibiotics to clear infection while maintaining supply. Binding or stopping feeds worsens engorgement; antifungals are ineffective. Early recognition prevents abscess formation and promotes rapid recovery.
SubChapter: Breast Infection Care
Q89. Answer: B
Explanation: Dysuria and frequency indicate urinary tract infection, common from catheterization or perineal trauma. Early culture and antibiotics prevent pyelonephritis. Diuresis causes increased output without burning; uterine infection presents with tenderness and lochia changes.
SubChapter: Urinary System Assessment
Q90. Answer: A
Explanation: Early gentle leg and ankle exercises enhance circulation, prevent thrombosis, and promote gradual recovery. Strenuous abdominal or weight activities strain healing tissues. Progressive increase in mobility supports safe rehabilitation and cardiovascular health postpartum.
SubChapter: Early Ambulation & Exercise Education
Q91. Answer: A
Explanation: Lactating women require about 500 additional daily calories and increased fluids to sustain milk supply and maternal health. Fluid restriction and nutrient deficiencies hinder production. Balanced nutrition supports recovery and infant growth simultaneously.
SubChapter: Lactation Nutrition Support
Q92. Answer: D
Explanation: Irritability and sleep disturbance beyond a few days may indicate emerging depression rather than transient blues. Early screening enables counseling or pharmacologic intervention before functional impairment develops, protecting maternal-infant bonding and safety.
SubChapter: Mental Health Screening Postpartum
Q93. Answer: A
Explanation: A firm, midline fundus at umbilical level shortly after birth is expected. Continued monitoring ensures progressive descent about 1 cm per day. A boggy or deviated fundus would require massage or voiding assistance.
SubChapter: Uterine Assessment Immediately Postpartum
Q94. Answer: A
Explanation: Cleaning from front to back prevents bacterial transfer from rectum to perineum, reducing infection risk. Scented wipes irritate healing tissue, and heat may increase swelling during early recovery. Consistent gentle cleansing supports comfort and wound healing.
SubChapter: Perineal Care and Hygiene Education
Q95. Answer: B
Explanation: Rapid pad saturation indicates hemorrhage, commonly from uterine atony. Immediate fundal massage restores tone and reduces bleeding. Documentation alone delays treatment, and rest or fever reduction is irrelevant until bleeding is controlled.
SubChapter: Hemorrhage Recognition and Response
Q96. Answer: B
Explanation: Engorgement occurs as milk transitions, causing firm and tender breasts for 24–48 hours. This is a normal physiologic response. Coldness suggests poor circulation; red streaks with fever indicate infection such as mastitis.

SubChapter: Breast Assessment and Education

Q97. Answer: B

Explanation: The "taking-in" phase occurs within the first 1–2 days, where mothers are passive, resting, and focused on their birth experience and newborn. Later, the "taking-hold" phase marks active learning and independence. Recognizing phases helps guide teaching.

SubChapter: Psychosocial Adaptation and Role Transition

Q98. Answer: D

Explanation: Warm compresses promote milk flow, and frequent nursing relieves pressure. Tight binding and fluid restriction worsen engorgement and discomfort. Supportive bras and complete emptying maintain comfort and lactation.

SubChapter: Lactation Management and Comfort

Q99. Answer: B

Explanation: Brief lochia increase after activity is common as pooled blood is expelled. Persistent heavy or malodorous bleeding indicates infection or retained tissue, while large clots suggest hemorrhage. Educating on normal variations prevents anxiety and ensures safety.

SubChapter: Lochial Assessment and Patient Teaching

Q100. Answer: B

Explanation: Fundal deviation commonly results from bladder distention, inhibiting uterine contraction and causing hemorrhage risk. The nurse should assist with voiding, then reassess tone. Other findings are expected at this stage of recovery.

SubChapter: Uterine and Bladder Assessment

Questions (101-200)

Q101. During postpartum teaching, the nurse explains that the best indicator of effective breastfeeding is:

A. The mother feels nipple tingling

B. The infant voids and stools adequately

C. Breasts remain firm after feeding

D. The mother hears swallowing only at start

Q102. A postpartum woman reports a headache and blurred vision 48 hours after delivery. What should the nurse suspect?

A. Sleep deprivation

B. Migraine recurrence

C. Normal fluid shifts

D. Postpartum preeclampsia

Q103. A nurse educates a patient on postpartum weight loss. Which statement demonstrates understanding?

A. "I will lose all my pregnancy weight within two weeks."

B. "Most fluid weight is lost in the first week."

C. "I should avoid exercise for six months."

D. "Breastfeeding prevents any weight loss."

Q104. A postpartum woman reports feeling dizzy after standing up quickly. Her blood pressure drops from 120/80 to 98/60 mmHg. The nurse explains this is likely due to:

A. Orthostatic hypotension

B. Postpartum hemorrhage

C. Infection

D. Hypoglycemia

Q105. Which finding indicates effective bladder emptying after delivery?

A. Voiding less than 100 mL every 2 hours

B. Absence of bladder distention with firm midline fundus

C. Fundus above umbilicus and deviated

D. Scant urine output with frequency

Q106. A nurse teaches a woman to recognize signs of infection after cesarean birth. Which statement shows understanding?

A. "I will call if my incision becomes red or drains fluid."

B. "Pain at the incision is always normal."

C. "I should remove steri-strips in two days."

D. "It's fine if the edges open slightly."

Q107. The nurse encourages early ambulation after birth primarily to prevent:

A. Constipation

B. Breast engorgement

C. Thromboembolism

D. Back pain

Q108. Which patient statement indicates the need for further teaching about breastfeeding nutrition?

A. "I'll drink an extra glass of water with each feeding."

B. "I can skip breakfast if I'm not hungry."

C. "I'll eat balanced meals with extra calories."

D. "I'll avoid alcohol completely."

Q109. A postpartum client reports urinary burning and urgency. The nurse's next action should be to:

A. Encourage increased fluid intake and notify the provider
B. Reassure her this is normal
C. Apply ice packs to the perineum
D. Limit oral fluids until symptoms improve

Q110. The nurse assesses emotional attachment during a postpartum visit. Which behavior best reflects bonding?

A. Ignoring the baby's cries
B. Maintaining eye contact and soothing the infant
C. Allowing staff to handle all feedings
D. Expressing disinterest in infant cues

Q111. A postpartum woman with an episiotomy asks about resuming exercise. The nurse should advise:

A. Begin heavy lifting after one week
B. Start light exercises when perineal pain subsides
C. Avoid movement for six weeks
D. Resume jogging immediately

Q112. A nurse is caring for a newborn who is 12 hours old and exhibits mild jitteriness, a weak cry, and a blood glucose level of 38 mg/dL. The mother had gestational diabetes controlled by diet during pregnancy. Which nursing intervention should the nurse perform first?

A. Notify the healthcare provider of the low glucose level
B. Initiate an IV infusion of 10% dextrose in water (D10W)
C. Feed the newborn with breast milk or formula immediately
D. Reassess the newborn's glucose level in 30 minutes

Q113. The nurse teaches a postpartum mother about warning signs. Which symptom requires immediate medical evaluation?

A. Mild afterpains during breastfeeding
B. Passage of tissue fragments with bleeding
C. Temporary mood swings
D. Light pink lochia

Q114. A nurse evaluates a woman's fundus two days postpartum and finds it soft and displaced to the right. What should the nurse do first?

A. Apply fundal massage and assist her to void.
B. Notify the healthcare provider immediately.
C. Increase her IV fluid rate.
D. Apply a warm compress to the abdomen.

Q115. Which postpartum finding requires immediate nursing intervention?

A. Fundus firm and midline
B. Scant lochia rubra on day 2
C. Temperature of 38.3 °C on day 3
D. Moderate afterpains during breastfeeding

Q116. Which comfort measure is most appropriate for hemorrhoid relief in a postpartum patient?

A. Ice packs followed by warm sitz baths
B. Direct massage of the area
C. Use of tight compression garments
D. Application of alcohol pads

Q117. A woman three days postpartum reports feeling "overwhelmed" and cries easily. What is the nurse's best response?

A. "You might need antidepressants immediately."

B. “These emotions are common and usually resolve soon.”
C. “You should avoid talking about your feelings.”
D. “It’s best to stay alone for a few days.”

Q118. The nurse instructs a postpartum patient with episiotomy care. Which statement indicates correct understanding?

A. “I’ll apply an antiseptic powder daily.”
B. “I’ll use a peri bottle after voiding to cleanse the area.”
C. “I’ll scrub the incision gently twice a day.”
D. “I’ll avoid changing pads frequently to reduce irritation.”

Q119. Which action supports lactation establishment during the early postpartum period?

A. Supplement formula after each feed
B. Breastfeed on demand, including nighttime
C. Limit feeding to 10 minutes per side
D. Delay feeding until milk comes in

Q120. The nurse assesses a postpartum patient’s emotional status. Which behavior suggests possible postpartum depression?

A. Expressing mild anxiety about infant care
B. Persistent sadness and loss of interest for three weeks
C. Fatigue relieved by rest
D. Occasional tearfulness the first few days

Q121. Which measure prevents thrombophlebitis in postpartum patients?

A. Encourage leg exercises and ambulation
B. Restrict movement for 24 hours
C. Apply cold packs to the calves routinely
D. Massage the legs firmly each shift

Q122. A postpartum woman experiences heavy bleeding with a firm uterus. The nurse suspects:

A. Uterine atony
B. Vaginal or cervical laceration
C. Retained placental fragments
D. Coagulation disorder

Q123. Which assessment finding is expected on the second postpartum day?

A. Fundus two centimeters below umbilicus
B. Lochia alba
C. Boggy uterus displaced to the right
D. Absence of lochia

Q124. When teaching about postpartum nutrition, the nurse emphasizes increasing intake of which nutrient for tissue repair?

A. Carbohydrates
B. Protein
C. Fats
D. Sodium

Q125. The nurse notes a patient’s uterus is soft after massage but becomes firm with breastfeeding. This finding indicates:

A. Need for additional oxytocin
B. Normal oxytocin release from nipple stimulation
C. Risk for infection
D. Retained placental fragments

Q126. A nurse instructs a postpartum woman about preventing constipation. Which statement shows understanding?
A. "I'll increase my fiber and fluid intake daily."
B. "I should avoid walking to prevent pain."
C. "Laxatives should be used every day."
D. "I'll reduce fluids to minimize bloating."
Q127. Which maternal response indicates strong infant attachment during the hospital stay?
A. Refers to the baby as "the infant"
B. Smiles and uses soft voice when holding the baby
C. Avoids touching the infant to prevent infection
D. Hands baby to nurse after each feed
Q128. A postpartum woman asks about resuming menstruation. Which statement is accurate for non-breastfeeding mothers?
A. "Your period usually returns within 6 to 10 weeks."
B. "It won't return for at least one year."
C. "You'll never ovulate before your first period."
D. "Bleeding will resume within one week."
Q129. A nurse observes the patient passing small clots and notes a foul odor from lochia. What is the priority action?
A. Document as normal rubra stage
B. Assess temperature and notify provider
C. Encourage ambulation
D. Apply cold compress to abdomen
Q130. Which postpartum activity best promotes venous circulation and reduces edema?
A. Elevating legs when sitting
B. Restricting fluids
C. Applying tight wraps to thighs
D. Prolonged standing
Q131. Which action helps a postpartum patient manage afterpains effectively?
A. Apply warmth and take mild analgesics as prescribed
B. Lie flat without movement
C. Avoid breastfeeding until pain subsides
D. Restrict fluids
Q132. The nurse counsels a breastfeeding mother with cracked nipples on care. Which practice is appropriate?
A. Wash nipples with soap and water after each feed
B. Air-dry nipples and apply purified lanolin
C. Cover nipples with plastic liners between feeds
D. Use alcohol pads for disinfection
Q133. A nurse evaluates a woman's understanding of danger signs. Which statement requires correction?
A. "Fever above 100.4°F should be reported."
B. "Heavy bright-red bleeding after the first week is normal."
C. "Foul-smelling discharge means infection."
D. "Pain, redness, or swelling in my leg is not normal."
Q134. A postpartum patient states her breasts feel heavy and painful on day 4. What nursing advice is most appropriate?
A. "Wear a supportive bra and express milk to comfort."

B. “Avoid feeding until pain subsides.”
C. “Apply ice before breastfeeding.”
D. “Restrict fluids to reduce fullness.”

Q135. A nurse reviews a postpartum woman’s chart and notes a hematocrit drop from 38% to 30% within 24 hours. What is the most likely cause?

A. Postpartum hemorrhage
B. Hemodilution
C. Laboratory error
D. Iron deficiency before delivery

Q136. Which finding suggests subinvolution of the uterus?

A. Fundus nonpalpable by two weeks
B. Lochia rubra persisting beyond 10 days
C. Firm midline uterus with scant lochia
D. Mild cramping after breastfeeding

Q137. The nurse assesses for postpartum depression during a home visit. Which statement is concerning?

A. “I feel sad and overwhelmed most of the time.”
B. “I’m tired but rest helps me feel better.”
C. “Sometimes I cry when I look at my baby, but I feel better later.”
D. “I’m nervous about doing things right.”

Q138. A woman complains of severe pain and swelling near the perineum 8 hours after birth. The fundus is firm and bleeding minimal. What should the nurse suspect?

A. Vulvar hematoma
B. Uterine atony
C. Endometritis
D. Retained placenta

Q139. A nurse evaluates urinary output after delivery. Which output indicates normal renal adaptation?

A. 100–200 mL/hr during first 24 hours
B. Less than 20 mL/hr consistently
C. No urine for 6 hours post-delivery
D. Continuous dark concentrated urine

Q140. Which statement by a postpartum patient indicates need for further teaching about sexual activity?

A. “We’ll use contraception when we resume intercourse.”
B. “It’s safe once lochia stops and healing is complete.”
C. “We can have sex as soon as I feel ready, even with bleeding.”
D. “Lubrication may be reduced while breastfeeding.”

Q141. The nurse teaches perineal care to prevent infection. Which instruction is appropriate?

A. Use warm water after each voiding
B. Apply talcum powder for dryness
C. Avoid pad changes unless saturated
D. Cleanse from back to front

Q142. The nurse observes excessive diaphoresis in a woman 24 hours postpartum. What is the correct interpretation?

A. Normal elimination of excess pregnancy fluid
B. Early sign of infection
C. Symptom of hypoglycemia

D. Result of hemorrhage

Q143. A postpartum patient complains of abdominal distention and absence of bowel movement for three days. The nurse should first:

A. Encourage ambulation and fluids
B. Administer a stimulant laxative immediately
C. Apply abdominal binder
D. Restrict dietary fiber

Q144. The nurse teaches a mother about preventing nipple soreness. Which instruction is most important?

A. Ensure the baby latches onto the areola, not just nipple
B. Limit feedings to five minutes
C. Wash breasts with soap after every feed
D. Use a pacifier between feeds

Q145. Which maternal finding on day 10 postpartum requires immediate attention?

A. Scant lochia alba
B. Return of bright-red bleeding
C. Nonpalpable uterus
D. Slight pelvic fullness

Q146. The nurse notes the patient's pulse is 55 bpm on day two postpartum. She is asymptomatic. What action should the nurse take?

A. Document as a normal physiologic finding
B. Notify the healthcare provider immediately
C. Increase IV fluids
D. Check for hemorrhage

Q147. A nurse is counseling a breastfeeding mother about returning to work. Which recommendation is appropriate?

A. Pump and store milk in sterile containers
B. Discontinue breastfeeding entirely
C. Replace daytime feedings with water
D. Avoid pumping to prevent leakage

Q148. Which vital sign change is a late indicator of postpartum hemorrhage?

A. Elevated pulse and decreasing blood pressure
B. Slight temperature increase
C. Bradycardia
D. Elevated blood pressure

Q149. The nurse observes that a new mother avoids holding her infant and appears withdrawn. What should the nurse do first?

A. Document behavior only
B. Force her to participate in feeding
C. Encourage discussion about her feelings and experiences
D. Inform her partner to take full responsibility

Q150. Which patient action helps prevent mastitis recurrence?

A. Alternate starting breast with each feeding
B. Restrict breastfeeding to once every 6 hours
C. Apply ice between every feeding only
D. Wear tight bras to prevent movement

Q151. During postpartum teaching, which advice helps prevent constipation?

A. Drink at least 2 liters of water daily

B. Avoid high-fiber foods
C. Delay ambulation until discharge
D. Take daily stimulant laxatives

Q152. The nurse provides discharge instructions to a cesarean birth patient. Which statement shows correct understanding?

A. "I will avoid lifting more than 10 pounds until cleared."
B. "It's safe to drive within a week."
C. "I can resume strenuous exercise immediately."
D. "I don't need to check the incision daily."

Q153. A nurse observes scant, odorless lochia on postpartum day eight. What is the correct interpretation?

A. Indicator of hemorrhage
B. Sign of retained placenta
C. Evidence of uterine infection
D. Normal transition to lochia alba

Q154. A postpartum patient complains of dizziness when standing. Her fundus is firm and lochia moderate. Which nursing action is most appropriate?

A. Assist her to change positions slowly and dangle legs first.
B. Report possible hemorrhage to the provider.
C. Administer oxygen immediately.
D. Place her in Trendelenburg position.

Q155. The nurse notes a postpartum woman's fundus is boggy and positioned above the umbilicus. What is the first nursing action?

A. Massage the fundus until firm.
B. Encourage oral fluids.
C. Notify the physician immediately.
D. Record as normal involution.

Q156. A nurse provides education to a woman experiencing afterpains. Which statement indicates understanding?

A. "They occur because my uterus is contracting back to normal."
B. "They mean my uterus isn't healing."
C. "They will last several weeks and worsen over time."
D. "I should stop breastfeeding to reduce them."

Q157. Which patient requires immediate evaluation?

A. Reports burning during urination
B. Reports night sweats and mild fatigue
C. Reports chills, fever, and foul-smelling lochia
D. Reports breast fullness on day 4

Q158. The nurse teaches a breastfeeding mother about nutrition. Which statement is correct?

A. "I need to drink an extra glass of water with each feeding."
B. "I should avoid dairy products completely."
C. "I must eat high-fat meals to increase milk."
D. "Skipping meals will not affect my supply."

Q159. Which finding indicates normal healing after cesarean birth on day five?

A. Incision edges well-approximated without redness
B. Purulent drainage at the incision site
C. Gaping incision edges with tenderness
D. Fever and chills present

Q160. A postpartum woman reports urinary frequency and burning. The nurse's priority action is to:
A. Obtain a urine specimen for culture.
B. Increase dietary iron intake.
C. Encourage pelvic floor exercises.
D. Apply a perineal ice pack.
Q161. Which instruction should the nurse give a patient with postpartum hemorrhoids?
A. Limit bowel movements to once daily.
B. Use cold applications only.
C. Avoid all activity until swelling decreases.
D. Increase fiber and fluids to prevent straining.
Q162. A postpartum woman states her perineum feels "tight and itchy" near the episiotomy site. What is the best response?
A. "That sensation often means the incision is healing."
B. "You probably have an infection."
C. "It indicates suture separation."
D. "You should stop cleaning the area."
Q163. A nurse provides discharge teaching for a breastfeeding mother. Which statement requires correction?
A. "I'll avoid tight bras to prevent blocked ducts."
B. "I can store expressed milk in the refrigerator for 4 days."
C. "I should apply alcohol before pumping."
D. "I'll wash my hands before handling milk containers."
Q164. Which patient behavior best reflects the "taking-hold" phase of maternal adaptation?
A. Passively relying on others for infant care
B. Seeking information and actively practicing infant care
C. Focusing primarily on herself and her needs
D. Detaching emotionally from the newborn
Q165. A postpartum woman experiences breast redness and fever. Which action should the nurse recommend?
A. Continue breastfeeding and start prescribed antibiotics.
B. Stop breastfeeding until symptoms resolve.
C. Apply ice constantly and avoid stimulation.
D. Bind breasts tightly.
Q166. Which statement by a new mother indicates proper understanding of postpartum exercise?
A. "I'll start with light walking once I feel comfortable."
B. "I'll wait six months to do any movement."
C. "I'll do abdominal crunches tomorrow."
D. "Exercise will increase my bleeding."
Q167. The nurse assesses a woman 10 days postpartum who reports increased bleeding after resuming housework. What should the nurse advise?
A. "Reduce activity and rest more frequently."
B. "That is an expected sign of recovery."
C. "You should increase iron supplements only."
D. "Ignore it unless you feel pain."
Q168. The nurse explains that lochia alba should appear by which postpartum day?
A. Day 2
B. Day 4
C. Day 10

D. Day 20

Q169. Which action reduces the risk of postpartum urinary retention?

A. Encourage voiding within 6 hours after birth.

B. Limit fluid intake to prevent distention.

C. Use a catheter routinely after every birth.

D. Delay voiding until urge returns.

Q170. Which postpartum behavior indicates impaired attachment?

A. Refers to the baby as "it" and avoids eye contact.

B. Smiles and talks to infant softly.

C. Responds promptly to baby's cries.

D. Expresses joy about bringing baby home.

Q171. A nurse educates a patient on signs of deep vein thrombosis. Which statement shows understanding?

A. "If my leg becomes red and painful, I'll call my provider."

B. "Swelling is normal after delivery."

C. "I'll massage my legs if they hurt."

D. "I'll keep my legs still to rest them."

Q172. Which teaching point is essential for postpartum women prescribed iron supplements?

A. Take with orange juice for better absorption.

B. Avoid vitamin C-rich foods.

C. Drink milk with the pill to reduce absorption.

D. Skip doses when stools are dark.

Q173. A postpartum woman reports burning and tenderness at her cesarean incision with yellow drainage. What should the nurse do?

A. Continue routine care.

B. Apply a dry dressing only.

C. Document as expected healing.

D. Notify the provider immediately.

Q174. A woman 12 hours postpartum reports constant perineal pressure and rectal pain. Fundus is firm and midline, but the perineum appears bruised and swollen. What should the nurse suspect?

A. Vaginal hematoma

B. Uterine atony

C. Endometritis

D. Episiotomy infection

Q175. Which patient statement requires further teaching about lochia?

A. "Lochia changes from red to brown to white."

B. "It's normal for the flow to increase after activity."

C. "I should report a foul odor or return to bright-red flow."

D. "Passing clots the size of lemons is expected."

Q176. A postpartum woman's temperature is 38 °C on day 1 but 37 °C on day 2. What is the correct nursing action?

A. Document as normal postpartum dehydration response.

B. Obtain blood cultures immediately.

C. Begin antibiotic therapy.

D. Restrict oral fluids.

Q177. A nurse evaluates breastfeeding effectiveness. Which observation confirms successful feeding?

A. Infant has six wet diapers daily.

B. Infant falls asleep within two minutes.

C. Breasts remain engorged after feeding.
D. Infant appears lethargic during feeding.

Q178. Which finding requires immediate follow-up on postpartum day 3?
A. Uterus firm, two cm below umbilicus
B. Lochia serosa pinkish-brown
C. Breasts warm and full
D. Red streak and tenderness on left calf

Q179. A postpartum woman with a perineal laceration asks when stitches will dissolve. What should the nurse reply?
A. "They usually dissolve within 2 to 3 weeks."
B. "They must be removed in 10 days."
C. "They will remain permanently."
D. "They dissolve within 24 hours."

Q180. Which instruction best prevents postpartum infection?
A. Change perineal pads frequently.
B. Use tampons for comfort.
C. Avoid handwashing before feeding.
D. Apply talcum powder to perineum.

Q181. A nurse assesses a patient reporting uterine tenderness and foul-smelling lochia five days postpartum. What condition does this suggest?
A. Endometritis
B. Mastitis
C. Retained urine
D. Normal healing

Q182. Which maternal vital-sign pattern suggests early postpartum hemorrhage?
A. Fever and chills
B. Bradycardia and hypertension
C. Normal vitals despite bleeding
D. Tachycardia and decreasing blood pressure

Q183. The nurse provides teaching about contraception while breastfeeding. Which statement shows understanding?
A. "I'll use progestin-only pills after six weeks."
B. "I'll take combined estrogen pills immediately."
C. "Breastfeeding alone prevents pregnancy completely."
D. "Barrier methods can't be used while nursing."

Q184. A postpartum woman's lochia changes from pink-brown to yellow-white on day 10. The nurse should:
A. Document this as normal progression.
B. Notify the provider.
C. Assess for retained fragments.
D. Begin antibiotics.

Q185. Which action should a nurse take for a woman reporting perineal pain unrelieved by medication?
A. Inspect perineum for hematoma or infection.
B. Reassure that pain is always normal.
C. Increase oral fluids only.
D. Encourage ambulation to reduce pain.

Q186. Which symptom requires emergency postpartum evaluation?

A. Breast tenderness day 3
B. Light pink lochia at two weeks
C. Mild cramps during feeding
D. Passing tissue fragments with bleeding

Q187. A nurse provides discharge instructions about postpartum exercise. Which statement indicates understanding?

A. “I’ll start pelvic exercises when my bleeding slows.”
B. “I’ll wait 6 months to begin any exercise.”
C. “I’ll avoid walking for 8 weeks.”
D. “I’ll begin crunches tomorrow.”

Q188. Which factor increases a postpartum woman’s risk for hemorrhage?

A. Prolonged labor and large baby
B. First-trimester pregnancy
C. Cesarean without complications
D. Breastfeeding within 30 minutes after birth

Q189. A postpartum woman complains of severe headache, blurred vision, and high blood pressure. What is the nurse’s first concern?

A. Postpartum preeclampsia
B. Migraine from fatigue
C. Dehydration
D. Sinus infection

Q190. A breastfeeding mother asks how to maintain supply after returning to work. Which guidance is best?

A. “Pump every 3–4 hours and store milk properly.”
B. “Skip pumping to reduce leaking.”
C. “Decrease water intake to slow production.”
D. “Use formula exclusively while working.”

Q191. Which nursing observation confirms uterine involution on day 7 postpartum?

A. Fundus tender and deviated
B. Fundus firm at umbilical level
C. Boggy uterus with heavy flow
D. Fundus halfway between symphysis and umbilicus

Q192. Which patient report on day 5 postpartum requires provider notification?

A. Fever 38.5 °C and chills
B. Soft breasts with colostrum
C. Mild cramping during feeding
D. Pink lochia with no odor

Q193. The nurse assesses a postpartum mother who expresses anxiety and doubts about caring for her baby. Which nursing action is most therapeutic?

A. Provide reassurance and offer hands-on teaching opportunities.
B. Assign care to family members only.
C. Tell her anxiety is abnormal and must stop.
D. Avoid discussing her concerns.

Q194. A postpartum woman reports feeling unusually sad and fatigued three weeks after birth. Which nursing response is most appropriate?

A. “These feelings may indicate postpartum depression; let’s contact your provider.”
B. “That’s normal; it happens to everyone.”
C. “Try resting more and it will pass.”

D. "Avoid visitors and focus on yourself."

Q195. The nurse observes a woman's fundus at the umbilicus and firm 6 hours postpartum. What should the nurse do?

A. Encourage ambulation immediately.
B. Massage the fundus vigorously.
C. Notify the healthcare provider.
D. Document the finding as normal.

Q196. A breastfeeding mother reports a burning sensation in both nipples and infant oral white patches. What is the likely cause?

A. Candida infection
B. Mastitis
C. Blocked milk duct
D. Normal adjustment

Q197. The nurse instructs a postpartum patient with hemorrhoids about bowel habits. Which statement shows understanding?

A. "I'll drink plenty of water and eat high-fiber foods."
B. "I should avoid fluids to prevent swelling."
C. "Straining will help empty my bowels completely."
D. "I'll use strong laxatives every day."

Q198. A postpartum patient's temperature is 37.9 °C, pulse 110 bpm, and lochia foul-smelling. What should the nurse suspect?

A. Endometritis
B. Normal dehydration
C. Breast engorgement
D. Bladder retention

Q199. A nurse provides education on postpartum exercises. Which activity is safe during the first week?

A. Aerobics classes
B. Sit-ups and crunches
C. Jogging and lifting
D. Deep-breathing and leg exercises

Q200. A woman experiences chills and shaking immediately after delivery. What is the nurse's best response?

A. Provide warm blankets and reassurance.
B. Call the provider for suspected infection.
C. Administer antibiotics immediately.
D. Begin cooling measures.

Answer key and Explanation (101-200)

Q101. Answer: B
Explanation: Consistent infant output (≥6 wet diapers and ≥3 stools daily) indicates adequate intake and successful breastfeeding. Tingling alone is subjective, and persistent firmness signals incomplete emptying. Continuous swallowing throughout feeding confirms good milk transfer.
SubChapter: Lactation Effectiveness Evaluation
Q102. Answer: D
Explanation: Severe headache and blurred vision may indicate elevated blood pressure due to postpartum preeclampsia. This requires immediate evaluation to prevent seizures or stroke. While fatigue and migraines are possible, hypertensive complications must be ruled out first.
SubChapter: Postpartum Complication Recognition
Q103. Answer: B
Explanation: Diuresis and hormonal shifts cause loss of 2–3 kg during the first week, but complete return takes several months. Safe exercise resumes gradually after clearance. Breastfeeding increases calorie use and supports healthy weight loss.
SubChapter: Nutrition and Physical Recovery
Q104. Answer: A
Explanation: Vasodilation and fluid shifts postpartum cause transient orthostatic hypotension. Gradual position changes prevent dizziness. Persistent hypotension with tachycardia, however, may signal hemorrhage or dehydration and requires evaluation.
SubChapter: Circulatory Adaptation and Safety Teaching
Q105. Answer: B
Explanation: A firm, midline fundus and absence of bladder distention indicate adequate emptying. Retention elevates and deviates the uterus, impeding contraction and increasing bleeding risk. Monitoring output and comfort ensures postpartum stability.
SubChapter: Elimination and Uterine Function
Q106. Answer: A
Explanation: Redness, drainage, or separation signal infection and require prompt medical evaluation. Incisional pain should gradually lessen, and strips should remain until removed professionally. Educating on early detection prevents sepsis and delayed healing.
SubChapter: Surgical Wound Care and Education
Q107. Answer: C
Explanation: Early ambulation enhances venous return and prevents thrombus formation, a major postpartum risk. It also promotes bowel motility but its chief benefit is circulation improvement. Safety support is essential during initial ambulation.
SubChapter: Circulatory Health Promotion
Q108. Answer: B
Explanation: Skipping meals reduces caloric intake and may impair milk production. Hydration and balanced nutrition are essential to sustain lactation and maternal recovery. Alcohol restriction is correct due to transfer into breast milk.
SubChapter: Nutrition During Lactation
Q109. Answer: A
Explanation: These symptoms suggest urinary tract infection; hydration dilutes urine and provider notification ensures timely antibiotic therapy. Restricting fluids worsens bacterial growth. Ice is for perineal swelling, not urinary discomfort.
SubChapter: Infection Prevention and Management
Q110. Answer: B

Explanation: Eye contact, soothing, and responsiveness demonstrate emotional bonding and maternal sensitivity. Lack of interest or avoidance behaviors may indicate adjustment difficulties requiring follow-up. Encouragement and education strengthen this developing connection.
SubChapter: Maternal–Infant Bonding Assessment
Q111. Answer: B
Explanation: Gentle activity, such as walking and pelvic tightening, may begin once discomfort resolves, supporting circulation and muscle tone. Strenuous exercise or lifting should wait until provider clearance, typically after six weeks.
SubChapter: Physical Recovery and Rehabilitation
Q112. Answer: C
Explanation: The newborn's blood glucose level (38 mg/dL) is below the normal range (≥45 mg/dL). The priority nursing action for asymptomatic or mildly symptomatic hypoglycemia in a term infant is early feeding to increase blood glucose. IV dextrose is reserved for newborns who are symptomatic or unable to feed. Reassessment and provider notification follow after the initial feeding intervention.
SubChapter: Newborn Assessment and Management of Physiologic Adaptations
Q113. Answer: B
Explanation: Passage of tissue fragments indicates possible retained placenta, leading to infection or hemorrhage if untreated. Mild cramping and emotional variability are expected. Prompt reporting ensures diagnostic evaluation and uterine evacuation if necessary.
SubChapter: Complication Recognition and Patient Education
Q114. Answer: A
Explanation: A soft, right-deviated fundus indicates bladder distention preventing contraction. The nurse should massage the fundus to stimulate tone, then help the patient void. Prompt correction prevents hemorrhage; notifying the provider or increasing fluids is unnecessary initially.
SubChapter: Uterine Assessment and Bladder Management
Q115. Answer: C
Explanation: Fever above 38 °C beyond the first 24 hours suggests infection such as endometritis. Early recognition ensures prompt antibiotic therapy. Firm fundus, light bleeding, and afterpains are expected findings during early postpartum recovery.
SubChapter: Infection Surveillance and Early Recognition
Q116. Answer: A
Explanation: Cold therapy reduces swelling and pain initially; warm sitz baths improve circulation and healing later. Massage and constrictive clothing worsen inflammation, while alcohol pads cause irritation. Consistent hygiene prevents infection and promotes comfort.
SubChapter: Perineal and Hemorrhoidal Care
Q117. Answer: B
Explanation: Emotional lability known as "baby blues" occurs within the first week due to hormonal shifts and fatigue. Support, rest, and reassurance help recovery. Persistent or worsening sadness warrants evaluation for depression.
SubChapter: Emotional Adaptation and Counseling
Q118. Answer: B
Explanation: Perineal irrigation with warm water after voiding prevents infection and promotes healing. Harsh scrubbing or infrequent pad changes increase irritation and bacterial growth. Powder use is discouraged because it interferes with tissue aeration.
SubChapter: Perineal Wound Hygiene
Q119. Answer: B

Explanation: Frequent on-demand feeding stimulates prolactin and oxytocin release, establishing milk supply. Supplementation and strict time limits interfere with lactation. Early initiation ensures successful breastfeeding and maternal-infant bonding.
SubChapter: Lactation Physiology and Education

Q120. Answer: B

Explanation: Persistent sadness, apathy, and impaired functioning lasting beyond two weeks signal postpartum depression requiring evaluation and therapy. Transient tearfulness or fatigue shortly after birth are typical adjustment responses.
SubChapter: Psychological Screening and Intervention

Q121. Answer: A

Explanation: Early ambulation and leg exercises enhance venous circulation and prevent clot formation. Massage risks embolus dislodgment, while inactivity increases stasis. Temperature therapy is unnecessary prophylactically.
SubChapter: Circulatory Health Promotion

Q122. Answer: B

Explanation: Persistent bright-red bleeding despite a firm uterus suggests trauma to genital tract tissues, commonly cervical or vaginal lacerations. Atony causes a boggy uterus, while retained fragments present with delayed bleeding and subinvolution.
SubChapter: Hemorrhage Etiology and Assessment

Q123. Answer: A

Explanation: The uterus descends about one centimeter per day, so by day two it should be two centimeters below the umbilicus. Early presence of alba or displacement indicates abnormal recovery.
SubChapter: Uterine Involution Monitoring

Q124. Answer: B

Explanation: Protein supports cell regeneration and tissue repair essential after childbirth. Carbohydrates and fats supply energy, while sodium excess causes fluid retention. Adequate protein intake enhances recovery and wound healing.
SubChapter: Postpartum Nutrition Education

Q125. Answer: B

Explanation: Nipple stimulation triggers oxytocin release, enhancing uterine contraction and involution—a normal physiologic reflex. Pharmacologic oxytocin isn't required unless tone remains poor. Persistent atony would require further evaluation.
SubChapter: Oxytocin Response and Uterine Physiology

Q126. Answer: A

Explanation: High fiber and fluids soften stools naturally and promote regular elimination. Walking aids bowel motility, while frequent laxatives risk dependence and dehydration. Proper diet and hydration maintain comfort.
SubChapter: Gastrointestinal Management and Teaching

Q127. Answer: B

Explanation: Smiling, affectionate tone, and gentle touch show emotional connection and secure bonding. Detachment, fear of contact, or minimal interaction suggests impaired attachment needing support.
SubChapter: Maternal–Infant Relationship Development

Q128. Answer: A

Explanation: In non-lactating women, menses generally returns between six and ten weeks postpartum. Ovulation may occur earlier; contraception is recommended. Extended amenorrhea is typical only in exclusive breastfeeding due to hormonal suppression.
SubChapter: Reproductive Function Education

Q129. Answer: B
Explanation: Foul odor and clot passage suggest infection or retained tissue. Checking temperature verifies systemic involvement, and prompt provider notification prevents progression to sepsis. Simple comfort measures are insufficient.
SubChapter: Infection Identification and Intervention
Q130. Answer: A
Explanation: Leg elevation assists venous return, decreasing edema and promoting comfort. Fluid restriction and prolonged standing worsen swelling, while constrictive garments impede circulation.
SubChapter: Circulatory Support and Education
Q131. Answer: A
Explanation: Heat therapy and mild analgesics relieve uterine contractions causing afterpains. Breastfeeding stimulates contractions that aid involution, so feeding should continue. Movement and hydration support recovery and pain control.
SubChapter: Pain Management and Comfort Measures
Q132. Answer: B
Explanation: Lanolin soothes and protects nipples, and air exposure promotes healing. Soap, alcohol, and occlusive materials cause irritation and delay recovery. Correct latch technique prevents recurrence.
SubChapter: Nipple Care and Breastfeeding Comfort
Q133. Answer: B
Explanation: Bright-red bleeding after the first week suggests abnormal subinvolution or retained fragments, not a normal finding. Other statements correctly identify warning signs requiring prompt medical attention.
SubChapter: Postpartum Danger Sign Education
Q134. Answer: A
Explanation: Engorgement from milk onset requires frequent feeding or expression to relieve pressure. A supportive bra reduces discomfort, while fluid restriction and feeding avoidance worsen engorgement. Ice before feeding delays let-down reflex and is not first-line.
SubChapter: Breast Engorgement Management
Q135. Answer: A
Explanation: A rapid hematocrit decline indicates significant blood loss from postpartum hemorrhage. Hemodilution changes are gradual, and pre-existing anemia would not produce such a sharp drop. Immediate assessment of bleeding and vital signs is essential.
SubChapter: Laboratory Interpretation in Postpartum Hemorrhage
Q136. Answer: B
Explanation: Persistent red lochia and a high fundal position beyond 10 days indicate subinvolution from retained fragments or infection. Normal involution results in a nonpalpable uterus by two weeks. Early recognition prevents chronic bleeding and infection.
SubChapter: Uterine Recovery Assessment
Q137. Answer: A
Explanation: Persistent sadness and loss of pleasure lasting beyond two weeks signal clinical depression needing referral. Temporary fatigue or mood swings are normal. Early detection reduces maternal morbidity and improves family adjustment.
SubChapter: Mental Health Screening and Support
Q138. Answer: A
Explanation: Localized perineal swelling with unrelieved pain despite firm uterus suggests a hematoma from vessel injury. Prompt assessment and surgical drainage may be required. Other causes would show uterine tenderness or heavy bleeding.
SubChapter: Trauma Identification and Management

Q139. Answer: A
Explanation: Postpartum diuresis removes excess fluid, leading to increased output within 24 hours. Oliguria or dark urine signals dehydration or obstruction. Monitoring ensures fluid balance and renal function recovery.
SubChapter: Fluid and Renal Adaptation
Q140. Answer: C
Explanation: Sexual activity before healing or while bleeding risks infection. Contraceptive use and recognizing lactation-related dryness show proper understanding. Early resumption disregards tissue recovery needs.
SubChapter: Sexual Health and Contraception Teaching
Q141. Answer: A
Explanation: Peri-bottle irrigation with warm water maintains hygiene and comfort, reducing infection risk. Powder and backward wiping introduce bacteria; frequent pad changes keep the area clean and dry.
SubChapter: Perineal Hygiene and Infection Prevention
Q142. Answer: A
Explanation: Postpartum diuresis and diaphoresis remove pregnancy-related fluid retention. It is normal unless accompanied by fever or tachycardia. Infection or hypovolemia produce additional systemic signs.
SubChapter: Physiologic Adaptation and Fluid Regulation
Q143. Answer: A
Explanation: Ambulation and hydration stimulate peristalsis and soften stool. Pharmacologic measures follow if conservative interventions fail. Fiber restriction worsens constipation; abdominal binders limit abdominal movement.
SubChapter: Gastrointestinal Function and Mobility
Q144. Answer: A
Explanation: Proper latch minimizes trauma by drawing the nipple deeply into the infant's mouth. Frequent cleaning or time restriction causes dryness and poor feeding. Effective positioning ensures comfort and successful breastfeeding.
SubChapter: Breastfeeding Technique Education
Q145. Answer: B
Explanation: Reappearance of bright-red bleeding indicates subinvolution or retained placental tissue. Normal progression includes alba discharge and nonpalpable uterus. Prompt evaluation prevents hemorrhage and infection.
SubChapter: Abnormal Bleeding Recognition
Q146. Answer: A
Explanation: Bradycardia of 50–70 bpm is normal due to increased stroke volume during early postpartum recovery. Only symptomatic changes require evaluation. Monitoring and documentation are appropriate.
SubChapter: Cardiovascular Adaptation Monitoring
Q147. Answer: A
Explanation: Expressing and storing breast milk safely allows continuation of breastfeeding after returning to work. Discontinuing or replacing with water disrupts nutrition. Proper storage preserves milk quality and supply.
SubChapter: Lactation Continuity Education
Q148. Answer: A
Explanation: Tachycardia with falling pressure signifies significant blood loss and compensatory shock response. Early recognition prevents hypovolemic collapse. Temperature and bradycardia are unrelated to acute bleeding.
SubChapter: Hemodynamic Assessment and Response

Q149. Answer: C

Explanation: Gentle communication allows expression of fears or anxiety, supporting bonding. Forced participation may increase distress. Early emotional support and observation guide further referral if depression or trauma is suspected.

SubChapter: Emotional Support and Bonding Facilitation

Q150. Answer: A

Explanation: Alternating breasts ensures complete emptying, reducing stasis and infection risk. Frequent feeding and gentle massage are essential. Tight garments and infrequent feeds contribute to obstruction and inflammation.

SubChapter: Mastitis Prevention and Breast Health

Q151. Answer: A

Explanation: Adequate hydration softens stools and aids bowel regularity. Fiber and ambulation further assist function. Regular laxative use causes dependence, and restriction increases discomfort. Hydration is the simplest, most effective preventive measure.

SubChapter: Bowel Management Education

Q152. Answer: A

Explanation: Limiting heavy lifting protects abdominal muscles and incision integrity. Driving or intense activity requires provider clearance. Daily inspection ensures early infection detection and promotes safe recovery.

SubChapter: Cesarean Recovery and Activity Teaching

Q153. Answer: D

Explanation: By one week postpartum, lochia typically lightens to yellow-white alba with minimal odor—an expected finding. Foul odor or persistent rubra suggests complications requiring evaluation.

SubChapter: Lochial Progression and Assessment

Q154. Answer: A

Explanation: Postpartum vascular changes can cause transient orthostatic hypotension; gradual position changes prevent falls. Firm uterus and moderate lochia rule out hemorrhage. Oxygen or Trendelenburg are unnecessary unless symptoms worsen.

SubChapter: Circulatory Adaptation and Safety Education

Q155. Answer: A

Explanation: A boggy, elevated fundus indicates uterine atony requiring immediate massage to stimulate contraction. This action prevents hemorrhage. If tone does not improve, the provider is notified for further management.

SubChapter: Hemorrhage Prevention and Uterine Tone

Q156. Answer: A

Explanation: Afterpains are caused by uterine contractions aiding involution. They intensify with breastfeeding due to oxytocin release and resolve within days. They indicate normal healing, not pathology.

SubChapter: Physiologic Recovery and Patient Education

Q157. Answer: C

Explanation: Fever, chills, and foul lochia indicate endometritis, a serious postpartum infection needing antibiotics. Urinary discomfort and engorgement are common; mild sweating reflects diuresis. Prompt recognition prevents sepsis.

SubChapter: Infection Detection and Management

Q158. Answer: A

Explanation: Adequate hydration supports milk production. Balanced nutrition and regular meals ensure nutrient supply for both mother and infant. Skipping meals or unbalanced diets may reduce milk quality and volume.

SubChapter: Lactation Nutrition Counseling
Q159. Answer: A
Explanation: Approximated incision edges without erythema or drainage confirm normal healing. Redness, separation, or drainage suggest infection requiring intervention. Continuous assessment ensures early detection of complications.
SubChapter: Postoperative Assessment and Wound Care
Q160. Answer: A
Explanation: Dysuria and frequency suggest urinary tract infection. A urine culture confirms diagnosis for targeted antibiotic therapy. Ice packs are for perineal swelling, not urinary symptoms.
SubChapter: Urinary Assessment and Infection Prevention
Q161. Answer: D
Explanation: Adequate fiber and hydration promote soft stools, reducing pressure and pain. Cold compresses may provide short-term relief, but dietary regulation prevents recurrence. Activity restriction worsens constipation.
SubChapter: Gastrointestinal Comfort and Preventive Care
Q162. Answer: A
Explanation: Mild itching or tightness reflects normal tissue healing and nerve regeneration. Infection would present with redness, drainage, or pain. Continued gentle cleansing prevents complications.
SubChapter: Perineal Healing Assessment
Q163. Answer: C
Explanation: Alcohol dries the skin and contaminates milk. Proper hand hygiene and safe storage ensure milk safety. Avoiding constrictive clothing prevents duct obstruction and mastitis.
SubChapter: Breastfeeding Hygiene and Storage Education
Q164. Answer: B
Explanation: During the “taking-hold” phase, mothers assume active responsibility for infant care and seek reassurance. The “taking-in” phase involves dependence, and emotional detachment suggests difficulty adapting.
SubChapter: Maternal Role Transition
Q165. Answer: A
Explanation: Mastitis treatment includes continued milk removal and antibiotics. Stopping feeds worsens engorgement and delays healing. Breast binding and constant cold compress hinder recovery.
SubChapter: Breast Infection Management
Q166. Answer: A
Explanation: Gentle walking aids circulation and recovery once tolerated. Strenuous exercise or long inactivity impedes healing and energy restoration. Gradual progression supports cardiovascular and muscular health.
SubChapter: Physical Rehabilitation and Education
Q167. Answer: A
Explanation: Increased bleeding after exertion suggests overactivity. Rest promotes healing and uterine recovery. Continuous bleeding or clots require evaluation, but mild flow increase signals need for decreased activity.
SubChapter: Activity Tolerance and Self-Care
Q168. Answer: C
Explanation: Lochia alba, yellow-white discharge, begins around day 10 and lasts several weeks as uterine healing progresses. Earlier changes reflect rubra or serosa stages. Monitoring helps identify infection or subinvolution.
SubChapter: Lochial Stage Progression
Q169. Answer: A

Explanation: Early voiding prevents bladder distention that interferes with uterine contraction. Fluid restriction and unnecessary catheterization increase infection risk. Encouraging toileting supports recovery.
SubChapter: Bladder Care and Uterine Function
Q170. Answer: A
Explanation: Avoidance behaviors, lack of eye contact, and impersonal language suggest emotional detachment or bonding difficulties. Early support and counseling help strengthen attachment and maternal confidence.
SubChapter: Emotional Bonding Assessment
Q171. Answer: A
Explanation: Redness, warmth, and pain in one leg indicate possible thrombosis needing prompt medical attention. Massage or inactivity risks embolism. Early ambulation and monitoring reduce occurrence.
SubChapter: Circulatory Complication Recognition
Q172. Answer: A
Explanation: Vitamin C enhances iron absorption. Milk and antacids inhibit uptake, and dark stools are normal. Consistent dosing ensures anemia recovery and energy restoration.
SubChapter: Nutritional Supplement Education
Q173. Answer: D
Explanation: Drainage, pain, and warmth indicate infection requiring medical evaluation and antibiotic therapy. Normal healing involves minimal tenderness and no discharge. Prompt reporting prevents wound dehiscence or sepsis.
SubChapter: Surgical Site Infection Management
Q174. Answer: A
Explanation: Severe, localized perineal pain with firm uterus and minimal bleeding indicates hematoma formation from vessel injury. Quick recognition allows drainage and pain relief. Atony causes soft uterus; infection produces fever and purulent drainage.
SubChapter: Perineal Trauma Assessment
Q175. Answer: D
Explanation: Large clots signal abnormal bleeding or retained fragments requiring evaluation. Color progression and slight increase after exertion are normal, while odor or heavy flow warrants provider notification.
SubChapter: Lochial Assessment and Education
Q176. Answer: A
Explanation: A mild, transient temperature rise during the first 24 hours reflects dehydration and exertion from labor. Normalization by day 2 confirms physiologic response, not infection. Hydration and rest suffice; antibiotics are unnecessary.
SubChapter: Vital Signs and Physiologic Adaptation
Q177. Answer: A
Explanation: Adequate urine output indicates sufficient intake and effective milk transfer. Persistent engorgement or lethargy suggests poor feeding technique requiring reassessment. Consistent output reflects maternal hydration and infant nutrition.
SubChapter: Lactation Effectiveness Monitoring
Q178. Answer: D
Explanation: Localized redness and tenderness suggest thrombophlebitis. Prompt evaluation prevents embolism. Other findings reflect normal recovery stages including involution, lochial transition, and milk onset.
SubChapter: Thromboembolic Complication Recognition
Q179. Answer: A

Explanation: Absorbable sutures typically dissolve as tissue heals over two to three weeks. No removal is needed. Removal or rapid dissolution times are inaccurate; healing progression determines comfort level.
SubChapter: Perineal Healing Education

Q180. Answer: A

Explanation: Frequent pad changes keep the perineum dry and decrease bacterial growth. Tampons introduce pathogens, while neglecting hand hygiene spreads infection. Proper hygiene promotes wound healing and maternal health.
SubChapter: Infection Prevention and Self-Care

Q181. Answer: A

Explanation: Foul odor, fever, and uterine tenderness indicate endometrial infection requiring antibiotics. Mastitis involves the breast; urinary retention affects elimination only. Early treatment prevents sepsis and fertility issues.
SubChapter: Postpartum Infection Recognition

Q182. Answer: D

Explanation: Tachycardia with hypotension signals volume loss and compensatory shock. Recognizing these subtle changes ensures timely intervention before critical deterioration. Other patterns indicate unrelated conditions.
SubChapter: Hemodynamic Assessment

Q183. Answer: A

Explanation: Progestin-only contraception is safe for lactation after six weeks. Estrogen decreases milk supply. Breastfeeding provides partial contraception but not full protection; barrier methods remain suitable options.
SubChapter: Contraceptive Education for Lactating Women

Q184. Answer: A

Explanation: Transition to lochia alba around day 10 reflects normal uterine healing. Abnormal persistence of rubra or foul odor would warrant evaluation. Proper documentation supports ongoing assessment.
SubChapter: Lochial Progression Monitoring

Q185. Answer: A

Explanation: Persistent, unrelieved perineal pain may indicate hematoma or infection. Assessment identifies complications requiring intervention. Simple reassurance or fluid adjustment does not address cause.
SubChapter: Pain Assessment and Follow-Up

Q186. Answer: D

Explanation: Tissue fragments suggest retained placenta, risking hemorrhage or infection. Early recognition allows uterine evacuation. Light lochia or engorgement are expected findings during recovery.
SubChapter: Complication Identification and Management

Q187. Answer: A

Explanation: Kegel and gentle walking can begin once lochia decreases and discomfort resolves, promoting tone and circulation. Extended inactivity delays recovery; strenuous exercise too early strains healing tissues.
SubChapter: Postpartum Rehabilitation Education

Q188. Answer: A

Explanation: Uterine overdistention and fatigue from prolonged labor predispose to atony and hemorrhage. Early breastfeeding promotes uterine contraction and is protective. Recognizing risk factors guides prevention.

SubChapter: Hemorrhage Risk Assessment

Q189. Answer: A

Explanation: Neurologic symptoms with hypertension indicate postpartum preeclampsia, requiring urgent evaluation to prevent seizures or stroke. Migraine or dehydration lack persistent hypertension.

SubChapter: Hypertensive Disorder Recognition

Q190. Answer: A

Explanation: Regular pumping maintains milk production and prevents engorgement. Proper storage ensures safe feeding. Skipping sessions or restricting fluids decreases supply.

SubChapter: Lactation Maintenance Counseling

Q191. Answer: D

Explanation: By one week postpartum, the uterus descends to mid-pelvic level, firm and midline. Elevated or boggy fundus suggests subinvolution or retention. Consistent assessment verifies normal progression.

SubChapter: Uterine Involution Monitoring

Q192. Answer: A

Explanation: Fever above 38 °C after 24 hours indicates infection. Early treatment with antibiotics prevents systemic spread. Other findings reflect normal adaptation to lactation and uterine involution.

SubChapter: Infection Surveillance

Q193. Answer: A

Explanation: Supportive reassurance and guided practice enhance maternal confidence and bonding. Avoidance or criticism worsens anxiety. Empowering education facilitates role transition and emotional stability.

SubChapter: Psychologic Support and Parenting Education

Q194. Answer: A

Explanation: Depressive symptoms lasting beyond two weeks suggest postpartum depression requiring evaluation and intervention. Early recognition ensures mental health support and prevents progression. Normal "baby blues" typically resolve within 10–14 days.

SubChapter: Mental Health Screening and Early Intervention

Q195. Answer: D

Explanation: Within the first 12 hours after delivery, the fundus should be firm and at or slightly above the umbilicus. Massage is unnecessary if tone is good. Ongoing monitoring ensures progressive descent over time.

SubChapter: Uterine Tone and Position Assessment

Q196. Answer: A

Explanation: Yeast infection (Candida) presents as nipple burning and infant thrush. Both mother and baby need antifungal treatment. Mastitis causes localized redness; blocked ducts create nodules. Hygiene and air-drying prevent recurrence.

SubChapter: Breastfeeding Complication Management

Q197. Answer: A

Explanation: Adequate hydration and fiber promote soft stools and prevent straining that worsens hemorrhoids. Laxative overuse causes dehydration and dependency. Proper diet and moderate activity enhance bowel regularity and comfort.

SubChapter: Gastrointestinal Health and Self-Care

Q198. Answer: A

Explanation: Fever, tachycardia, and offensive lochia indicate endometrial infection. Immediate antibiotic therapy prevents progression to sepsis. Dehydration causes mild fever without odor; engorgement or urinary issues lack uterine tenderness.

SubChapter: Postpartum Infection Identification

Q199. Answer: D
Explanation: Gentle leg and breathing exercises enhance circulation and lung expansion, preventing thrombosis. Strenuous activities strain healing tissues and delay recovery. Gradual progression promotes safe rehabilitation.
SubChapter: Physical Rehabilitation Education
Q200. Answer: A
Explanation: Post-delivery chills result from vascular and hormonal shifts, not infection. Comfort measures such as warm blankets and reassurance suffice. Persistent fever or uterine tenderness would warrant further assessment.
SubChapter: Immediate Postpartum Physiologic Response

Questions (201-300)

Q201. Which nursing intervention promotes bonding between mother and newborn?

A. Encourage skin-to-skin contact soon after birth.
B. Delay infant contact until day two.
C. Keep baby in nursery for rest periods.
D. Limit touching to prevent overstimulation.

Q202. The nurse teaches a postpartum woman with a cesarean incision about signs of infection. Which statement requires further teaching?

A. "Redness and drainage around my incision are normal."
B. "I'll report any fever or foul-smelling drainage."
C. "I'll keep the incision clean and dry."
D. "I'll avoid tight clothing over the incision."

Q203. A woman 3 days postpartum has cracked nipples and reports pain while breastfeeding. What should the nurse assess first?

A. Milk supply volume
B. Mother's hydration status
C. Maternal diet
D. Infant's latch and positioning

Q204. Which factor increases risk of postpartum infection?

A. Prolonged rupture of membranes
B. Early ambulation
C. Breastfeeding within first hour
D. Voiding within 2 hours of birth

Q205. Which symptom should be reported immediately to the provider?

A. Heavy bright-red bleeding after day 7
B. Fatigue relieved by rest
C. Pink lochia at day 5
D. Mild afterpains during feeding

Q206. Which nursing instruction aids in preventing postpartum urinary tract infection?

A. Void frequently and completely.
B. Limit oral fluids.
C. Delay urination until urge is strong.
D. Avoid cleansing after voiding.

Q207. The nurse provides discharge teaching to a woman with a cesarean incision. Which instruction is correct?

A. "Report redness, swelling, or drainage from the incision."
B. "Avoid showering until your follow-up visit."
C. "You may lift objects over 20 pounds."
D. "You can drive once discharged."

Q208. Which maternal finding at two weeks postpartum requires evaluation?

A. No perineal discomfort
B. Nonpalpable uterus
C. Small amount of yellow lochia
D. Persistent lochia rubra

Q209. Which patient behavior reflects positive maternal adaptation?

A. Expresses joy when holding her infant
B. Avoids touching the baby

C. Shows no interest in feeding
D. Refers to infant as “it”

Q210. The nurse instructs a patient about Kegel exercises. Which statement shows understanding?
A. “I’ll tighten my pelvic muscles for 10 seconds, 10 times a day.”
B. “I’ll perform them while urinating each time.”
C. “I should avoid them until 6 months postpartum.”
D. “They strengthen my abdominal muscles.”

Q211. A postpartum woman reports feeling dizzy and lightheaded 4 days after birth. Her hemoglobin is 8 g/dL. What is the most likely cause?
A. Postpartum anemia
B. Dehydration
C. Infection
D. Hypertension

Q212. Which assessment finding suggests normal breast adaptation in a breastfeeding mother?
A. Localized redness and swelling
B. Nipples cracked and bleeding
C. Breasts soft and non-tender throughout
D. Breasts firm, warm, and slightly tender on day 3

Q213. A postpartum nurse notices a new mother crying while saying she feels like a failure. What should the nurse do?
A. Listen empathetically and provide reassurance that these feelings are common.
B. Ignore the behavior to avoid embarrassment.
C. Tell her to rest more and stop crying.
D. Inform family to leave her alone.

Q214. A postpartum patient reports chills and a temperature of 38.7 °C on day three. Lochia is foul-smelling, and the uterus is tender. What should the nurse suspect?
A. Endometritis
B. Mastitis
C. Cystitis
D. Normal recovery

Q215. Which teaching point should the nurse emphasize to prevent constipation in the postpartum period?
A. Increase dietary fiber and water intake daily.
B. Avoid fruits and vegetables for one week.
C. Restrict fluids until lochia decreases.
D. Delay ambulation to rest.

Q216. A nurse assesses a woman 10 days postpartum with heavy red bleeding. The uterus is soft and above the symphysis. What should the nurse do first?
A. Encourage oral fluids only.
B. Apply an abdominal binder.
C. Document findings as normal.
D. Massage the fundus firmly.

Q217. A postpartum woman reports urinary urgency and burning. Which action should the nurse take first?
A. Obtain a clean-catch urine specimen for culture.
B. Encourage increased dietary iron intake.
C. Provide an ice pack to the perineum.
D. Reassure that symptoms are normal.

Q218. A mother on postpartum day four complains of painful, reddened breast area with fever. Which nursing advice is best?

A. Continue breastfeeding and begin prescribed antibiotics.
B. Stop breastfeeding until the pain subsides.
C. Apply ice constantly and bind the breasts.
D. Avoid pumping until healed.

Q219. Which maternal behavior demonstrates positive parent–infant attachment?

A. Smiles and talks softly to the infant during feeding.
B. Avoids touching the baby to prevent spoiling.
C. Asks the nurse to keep baby in nursery overnight.
D. Shows no interest in learning infant cues.

Q220. A patient's lochia changes from pink to yellow-white by day 10 postpartum. What does this finding indicate?

A. Subinvolution of the uterus.
B. Infection requiring antibiotics.
C. Retained placental fragments.
D. Normal healing process.

Q221. The nurse assesses a postpartum patient with a firm fundus but bright-red bleeding. Which condition is most likely?

A. Vaginal or cervical laceration
B. Uterine atony
C. Retained placenta
D. Endometritis

Q222. A postpartum mother complains of persistent sadness and loss of interest in daily activities four weeks after birth. Which nursing action is appropriate?

A. Refer her for evaluation of postpartum depression.
B. Encourage more rest and reassurance only.
C. Explain it's part of normal adjustment.
D. Suggest she stop breastfeeding.

Q223. Which nursing teaching helps prevent perineal infection after delivery?

A. Cleanse front to back after urination.
B. Use tampons instead of pads.
C. Apply powder to the perineum.
D. Avoid perineal cleansing for two days.

Q224. A postpartum woman experiences heavy bleeding with clots one week after discharge. What should the nurse instruct her to do?

A. Resume normal activity.
B. Rest and observe for another day.
C. Seek immediate medical evaluation.
D. Increase fluid intake only.

Q225. A breastfeeding woman asks when her menses will return. Which statement is correct?

A. "If you exclusively breastfeed, your period may not return for several months."
B. "Your period will return within two weeks."
C. "Breastfeeding has no effect on menstruation."
D. "You will never menstruate while lactating."

Q226. A postpartum nurse observes that a patient avoids looking at or holding her infant. What should the nurse do first?

A. Engage the mother in gentle conversation about her feelings.

B. Report immediately to psychiatric services.
C. Force her to hold the baby.
D. Ignore the behavior.

Q227. A postpartum woman asks about resuming sexual activity. Which teaching is correct?
A. "It's safe once lochia stops and healing is complete, usually by six weeks."
B. "You may resume immediately after discharge."
C. "Wait at least six months."
D. "Avoid contraception if breastfeeding."

Q228. The nurse teaches a postpartum woman to recognize infection signs. Which symptom should she report?
A. Fatigue after caring for infant
B. Mild breast fullness day 3
C. Small yellow lochia day 10
D. Fever and foul-smelling discharge

Q229. A nurse evaluates fundal height two days after delivery. Which finding is normal?
A. Two centimeters below the umbilicus
B. At the umbilical level
C. Four centimeters above the umbilicus
D. Not palpable

Q230. Which intervention is most effective in relieving breast engorgement for a breastfeeding mother?
A. Feed frequently and apply warm compresses before feeding.
B. Restrict fluids to reduce swelling.
C. Skip feedings for several hours.
D. Apply tight bandages around breasts.

Q231. A postpartum woman complains of severe calf pain and swelling. What should the nurse do first?
A. Notify the healthcare provider immediately.
B. Encourage ambulation.
C. Massage the calf to relieve tension.
D. Apply warm compresses without assessment.

Q232. A mother on postpartum day 2 reports frequent urination of large volumes. How should the nurse interpret this finding?
A. Evidence of dehydration.
B. Early symptom of diabetes.
C. Sign of urinary infection.
D. Normal diuresis eliminating excess pregnancy fluid.

Q233. The nurse assesses a postpartum woman's incision that is red, warm, and draining pus. What should the nurse do next?
A. Notify the healthcare provider for possible antibiotics.
B. Clean with alcohol and cover tightly.
C. Document as normal inflammation.
D. Apply heat and ignore drainage.

Q234. A postpartum patient complains of severe perineal pain unrelieved by medication; the nurse notes firm uterus and slight bulge near the perineum. What condition is suspected?
A. Vaginal hematoma
B. Uterine atony
C. Endometritis

D. Episiotomy infection

Q235. The nurse teaches a mother with a cesarean incision about activities at home. Which statement shows understanding?

A. "I'll avoid lifting anything heavier than my baby for six weeks."

B. "I can drive as soon as I feel ready."

C. "I'll take daily bubble baths for comfort."

D. "Stairs are fine immediately after discharge."

Q236. A postpartum woman's pulse is 52 bpm on day 2 with stable blood pressure and no distress. What should the nurse do?

A. Begin cardiac monitoring.

B. Report bradycardia to provider immediately.

C. Document this normal finding.

D. Administer oxygen.

Q237. Which teaching point helps a breastfeeding mother prevent nipple soreness?

A. Ensure baby latches onto both nipple and areola.

B. Limit feedings to five minutes per side.

C. Clean nipples with alcohol after each feed.

D. Use tight bras for support.

Q238. A nurse assesses a postpartum client complaining of severe abdominal pain and minimal lochia. The uterus is firm and displaced to the right. What should the nurse do first?

A. Assist her to void.

B. Massage the fundus.

C. Administer analgesics.

D. Increase fluid restriction.

Q239. Which maternal statement indicates successful coping with postpartum role change?

A. "I'm learning to balance my needs and the baby's schedule."

B. "I let everyone else handle the baby."

C. "I feel no emotional connection to my infant."

D. "I regret becoming a mother."

Q240. A nurse counsels a postpartum woman prescribed iron supplements. Which statement needs correction?

A. "I'll take iron with orange juice."

B. "Dark stools are expected."

C. "I'll take it with milk to prevent nausea."

D. "I'll continue for several months."

Q241. Which nursing instruction aids in preventing thrombophlebitis after cesarean birth?

A. Encourage early ambulation and leg exercises.

B. Keep patient in bed for 48 hours.

C. Apply tight abdominal binders continuously.

D. Restrict fluids to reduce edema.

Q242. The nurse teaches perineal care to a woman with second-degree laceration. Which practice is correct?

A. Use warm peri-bottle cleansing after each void.

B. Avoid washing for 24 hours.

C. Apply powder for dryness.

D. Use tampons to absorb discharge.

Q243. A postpartum mother states, "I'm afraid I'll hurt my baby accidentally." How should the nurse respond?

A. Acknowledge her fear and provide reassurance with teaching.
B. Tell her those fears are irrational.
C. Leave the infant with relatives.
D. Ignore her statement.

Q244. A postpartum client with episiotomy complains of burning during urination. What should the nurse assess for first?

A. Breast engorgement.
B. Kidney stones.
C. Infection or laceration irritation.
D. Hemorrhoids.

Q245. Which symptom on day 5 requires immediate evaluation?

A. Sudden bright-red bleeding after previous serosa stage.
B. Mild uterine cramping during nursing.
C. Fatigue after nighttime feeding.
D. Slight breast warmth.

Q246. A breastfeeding mother reports nipple pain and white plaques in the infant's mouth. What teaching should the nurse provide?

A. Treat both mother and infant for Candida infection.
B. Stop breastfeeding until symptoms disappear.
C. Use topical alcohol wipes.
D. Discard all expressed milk.

Q247. Which assessment finding indicates healthy emotional adjustment?

A. Expresses joy and confidence caring for infant.
B. Avoids participation in infant feeding.
C. Refuses to rest and overexerts herself.
D. Shows persistent tearfulness.

Q248. A postpartum patient complains of increased pain and swelling at the incision site with fever. What is the nurse's first action?

A. Record as normal inflammation.
B. Reinforce dressing tightly.
C. Apply warm compresses without assessment.
D. Notify the healthcare provider immediately.

Q249. Which advice promotes adequate lactation for a nursing mother?

A. Feed every 2–3 hours and maintain hydration.
B. Restrict fluids to prevent leakage.
C. Skip nighttime feedings.
D. Avoid high-protein foods.

Q250. A postpartum nurse notes patient anxiety, poor concentration, and insomnia two weeks after delivery. What should the nurse suspect?

A. Postpartum depression
B. Normal fatigue
C. Endometritis
D. Thyroid dysfunction

Q251. The nurse advises a woman with hemorrhoids to use which comfort measure?

A. Sitz baths several times daily.
B. Ice continuously for 24 hours.
C. Avoid fluids to reduce swelling.
D. Insert rectal suppositories routinely.

Q252. Which maternal assessment indicates successful uterine involution on day 5 postpartum?
A. Fundus nonpalpable.
B. Fundus boggy and above umbilicus.
C. Fundus tender and deviated.
D. Fundus firm and midway between symphysis and umbilicus.
Q253. The nurse observes a postpartum patient trembling and emotional while discussing her birth experience. What is the best nursing response?
A. Listen actively and validate her feelings.
B. Change subject to distract her.
C. Tell her to rest and stop crying.
D. Minimize importance of her concerns.
Q254. Which assessment finding in a term newborn indicates a need for immediate respiratory support?
A. Nasal flaring
B. Irregular respirations during sleep
C. Occasional sneezing
D. Brief acrocyanosis
Q255. The nurse notes a heart rate of 85 bpm in a quiet newborn. What should the nurse do first?
A. Stimulate the infant gently
B. Begin chest compressions
C. Call for the neonatal resuscitation team
D. Increase environmental temperature
Q256. Which assessment finding requires notifying the provider immediately?
A. Slight head molding
B. Temperature of 97.2°F (36.2°C)
C. Absent femoral pulses
D. Overlapping cranial sutures
Q257. A newborn's blood glucose is 36 mg/dL. What is the appropriate initial intervention?
A. Administer 10% dextrose IV
B. Feed the infant breast milk or formula
C. Notify the provider immediately
D. Repeat glucose in 6 hours
Q258. Which characteristic best describes a normal newborn respiratory pattern?
A. Rate 20–30 breaths/min
B. Periodic breathing with brief pauses under 10 seconds
C. Grunting during expiration
D. Sustained chest retractions
Q259. During a newborn exam, a single umbilical artery is observed. What action should the nurse anticipate?
A. Discharge teaching on cord care
B. Apply antibiotic ointment
C. Perform additional cord cleaning
D. Notify provider for renal ultrasound order
Q260. Which finding is typical in a healthy full-term infant at 24 hours old?
A. Absent rooting reflex
B. Positive Babinski reflex
C. Jaundice extending to the legs
D. Fixed dilated pupils

Q261. The nurse observes jitteriness in a newborn. What should be assessed first?
A. Serum calcium
B. Blood glucose
C. Body temperature
D. Bilirubin level
Q262. When performing a head-to-toe exam, which step should the nurse perform last?
A. Palpate abdomen
B. Assess heart and lungs
C. Inspect genitalia
D. Examine eyes and mouth
Q263. A 1-day-old newborn shows a temperature of 95.5°F (35.3°C). Which intervention is priority?
A. Feed immediately
B. Place under a radiant warmer
C. Notify provider for sepsis workup
D. Swaddle and observe
Q264. Which finding indicates normal cardiovascular transition after birth?
A. Persistent cyanosis
B. Functional closure of the ductus arteriosus
C. Murmur with decreased femoral pulses
D. Central cyanosis on crying
Q265. Which newborn finding would the nurse document as abnormal?
A. Irregular heart rate that varies with respirations
B. Soft systolic murmur at left sternal border
C. Persistent tachycardia >180 bpm at rest
D. Acrocyanosis at 10 minutes after birth
Q266. Which action promotes thermoregulation immediately after birth?
A. Bathe the newborn promptly
B. Dry and place skin-to-skin with mother
C. Apply cool blankets
D. Delay drying until stable
Q267. Which sign suggests respiratory distress syndrome in a preterm newborn?
A. Grunting and sternal retractions
B. Periodic breathing
C. Sneezing and hiccups
D. Acrocyanosis
Q268. The nurse notes a large cephalohematoma. What complication should be monitored?
A. Hypoglycemia
B. Hyperbilirubinemia
C. Hypothermia
D. Hypocalcemia
Q269. Which newborn reflex assists with feeding?
A. Moro
B. Palmar grasp
C. Rooting
D. Stepping
Q270. A newborn's skin shows lanugo and vernix. Which interpretation is correct?
A. Postterm infant
B. Premature infant

C. Term infant
D. Pathologic condition

Q271. When assessing newborn pain, which behavioral cue is most reliable?
A. Yawning
B. Rhythmic sucking
C. Brow bulge and cry
D. Rooting reflex

Q272. The nurse notes a caput succedaneum. Which description applies?
A. Localized swelling crossing suture lines
B. Blood collection under periosteum
C. Bruising limited to parietal area
D. Hemorrhage causing skull asymmetry

Q273. Which intervention supports successful transition to extrauterine life immediately after delivery?
A. Delay drying to maintain vernix
B. Clear airway only if obstruction noted
C. Routinely suction mouth and nose
D. Initiate feeding before thermal stabilization

Q274. Which newborn assessment should be prioritized immediately after birth?
A. Skin turgor
B. Airway patency
C. Reflex response
D. Umbilical cord color

Q275. A term infant has a respiratory rate of 70 with mild retractions. What is the likely cause?
A. Transient tachypnea of the newborn
B. Persistent pulmonary hypertension
C. Respiratory distress syndrome
D. Meconium aspiration syndrome

Q276. Which finding most strongly indicates neonatal infection?
A. Mild jaundice
B. Temperature instability
C. Pink mucous membranes
D. Acrocyanosis

Q277. Which statement best describes a normal newborn heart sound?
A. Split S2 during inspiration
B. Continuous murmur through cycle
C. Fixed S2 splitting unaffected by breathing
D. Harsh systolic murmur over aortic area

Q278. Which measurement reflects accurate newborn growth assessment?
A. Weight only
B. Head circumference and length
C. Weight, length, and head circumference
D. Chest circumference alone

Q279. A newborn's hematocrit is 68 %. Which risk should the nurse anticipate?
A. Anemia
B. Polycythemia-related hyperviscosity
C. Bleeding disorder
D. Infection

Q280. Which action best prevents heat loss via evaporation?
A. Warm room environment
B. Dry newborn immediately after birth
C. Cover head with cap after one hour
D. Avoid metal scale contact
Q281. During assessment, a neonate's axillary temperature is 97°F (36.1°C). Which nursing action is most appropriate?
A. Place under radiant warmer and recheck in 30 minutes
B. Administer glucose gel immediately
C. Begin antibiotic therapy
D. Delay intervention and observe
Q282. Which skin finding is benign in newborns?
A. Petechiae on trunk
B. Erythema toxicum rash
C. Cyanosis of lips and tongue
D. Jaundice within 12 hours
Q283. Which reflex should disappear first during normal development?
A. Moro
B. Stepping
C. Palmar grasp
D. Rooting
Q284. Which newborn has the highest risk for hypoglycemia?
A. Term AGA infant
B. Postterm infant
C. Infant of diabetic mother
D. Preterm AGA infant
Q285. A newborn vomits green fluid and shows abdominal distention. What should the nurse suspect?
A. Pyloric stenosis
B. Necrotizing enterocolitis
C. Bowel obstruction
D. Gastroesophageal reflux
Q286. Which finding requires prompt neonatal provider evaluation?
A. Scaphoid abdomen with respiratory distress
B. Active bowel sounds
C. Umbilical cord drying at 2 days
D. Slight abdominal protuberance after feeding
Q287. What is the expected output pattern for a hydrated term infant by day 3?
A. 1 wet diaper per day
B. 3–4 wet diapers daily
C. 6 or more wet diapers daily
D. Variable output until week 2
Q288. A 24-hour-old infant's bilirubin is 10 mg/dL. Which action is appropriate?
A. Begin phototherapy immediately
B. Encourage frequent feedings and monitor levels
C. Discontinue breastfeeding
D. No intervention required
Q289. Which assessment indicates effective oxygenation in a newborn on room air?
A. Central cyanosis

B. Pink color with $SpO_2 > 95$ %
C. $SpO_2 < 90$ % after 5 minutes
D. Peripheral cyanosis with crying

Q290. What is the nurse's best action for a newborn exhibiting grunting and nasal flaring?
A. Apply oxygen and notify provider immediately
B. Feed to increase energy stores
C. Swaddle and observe for resolution
D. Delay intervention for 30 minutes

Q291. Which assessment finding in a newborn suggests hypocalcemia?
A. High-pitched cry and tremors
B. Lethargy and poor suck
C. Flushed skin and rapid pulse
D. Low temperature and bradycardia

Q292. Which assessment finding requires follow-up before discharge?
A. Heart murmur persisting after 48 hours
B. Epstein pearls on palate
C. Transitory acrocyanosis
D. Erythema toxicum rash

Q293. Which action should the nurse take when a newborn fails hearing screen in both ears?
A. Repeat screen immediately after feeding
B. Document and discharge without concern
C. Schedule repeat screen in 2 weeks and notify parents
D. Begin antibiotic therapy

Q294. Which initial assessment confirms adequate neonatal perfusion?
A. Capillary refill under 3 seconds
B. Acrocyanosis beyond 10 minutes
C. Cool extremities with pink trunk
D. Systolic BP < 50 mm Hg

Q295. A term infant's respiratory rate is 32 and lungs are clear. What is the nurse's action?
A. Notify provider
B. Document as normal finding
C. Initiate supplemental oxygen
D. Delay feeding

Q296. Which finding suggests hypothermia rather than infection?
A. Lethargy and bradycardia
B. Temperature instability with tachypnea
C. Mottled skin and poor feeding
D. Apnea and pallor

Q297. During assessment, a soft murmur appears only during crying. What does this indicate?
A. Transitional physiologic flow murmur
B. Patent ductus arteriosus
C. Ventricular septal defect
D. Aortic stenosis

Q298. Which assessment finding is expected in a term infant 12 hours after birth?
A. Strong cry and active movement
B. Abdominal distention and vomiting
C. Intercostal retractions
D. Cyanotic nail beds

Q299. A 3-day-old infant shows weight loss of 8 %. What is the nurse's response?
A. Encourage frequent feeds and monitor
B. Initiate IV fluids
C. Report as abnormal dehydration
D. Start formula supplementation immediately
Q300. Which assessment confirms adequate neuromuscular tone in a newborn?
A. Limp posture at rest
B. Flexed extremities and spontaneous movement
C. Asymmetric Moro response
D. Poor sucking effort

Answer key and Explanation (201-300)

Q201. Answer: A
Explanation: Early skin-to-skin contact enhances maternal oxytocin release and emotional connection, supporting breastfeeding and attachment. Delays or separation hinder bonding and may increase maternal anxiety.
SubChapter: Maternal–Infant Bonding Promotion
Q202. Answer: A
Explanation: Redness and drainage signify infection and require prompt medical attention. Clean, dry care and loose clothing promote healing. Early reporting prevents systemic spread.
SubChapter: Surgical Wound Care and Infection Prevention
Q203. Answer: D
Explanation: Improper latch is the primary cause of nipple trauma. Correcting infant positioning relieves pain and promotes effective feeding. Milk supply and diet contribute secondarily but are not initial causes.
SubChapter: Breastfeeding Technique Evaluation
Q204. Answer: A
Explanation: Extended membrane rupture allows bacterial entry, heightening infection risk. Early breastfeeding and voiding facilitate recovery and reduce complications. Awareness of risk factors ensures proactive monitoring.
SubChapter: Infection Risk Identification
Q205. Answer: A
Explanation: Return of heavy bright-red flow indicates subinvolution or retained tissue, risking hemorrhage. Normal progression includes fading discharge and mild cramps. Prompt reporting ensures intervention.
SubChapter: Abnormal Bleeding Recognition
Q206. Answer: A
Explanation: Regular, complete voiding clears bacteria and prevents stasis. Adequate fluids and perineal hygiene further reduce risk. Restricting fluids or delaying urination increases infection likelihood.
SubChapter: Urinary System Care and Prevention
Q207. Answer: A
Explanation: Redness, drainage, or swelling suggest infection and must be reported. Gentle showering is allowed after 48 hours. Heavy lifting and driving should wait until medical clearance.
SubChapter: Cesarean Postoperative Education
Q208. Answer: D
Explanation: Rubra beyond one week indicates subinvolution or retained products, requiring assessment. A nonpalpable uterus and yellow lochia signify normal healing.
SubChapter: Uterine Involution Monitoring
Q209. Answer: A
Explanation: Joyful interaction and affectionate behavior demonstrate healthy bonding. Avoidance, disinterest, or depersonalization suggest delayed attachment needing support and evaluation.
SubChapter: Maternal Role and Bonding Assessment
Q210. Answer: A
Explanation: Regular Kegel exercises strengthen pelvic floor muscles, improving bladder control. Doing them during urination is only for identification of the muscle group, not routine practice. Early initiation supports recovery.
SubChapter: Pelvic Floor Rehabilitation Education
Q211. Answer: A

Explanation: Hemoglobin of 8 g/dL indicates anemia from blood loss. Symptoms include dizziness and fatigue. Iron supplementation and dietary improvement are key to recovery. Dehydration or hypertension would present differently.
SubChapter: Hematologic Assessment and Care

Q212. Answer: D

Explanation: Engorgement during milk onset is normal, lasting 24–48 hours. Persistent pain, cracking, or redness indicates complications. Monitoring ensures timely support and comfort measures.
SubChapter: Lactation Physiology Assessment

Q213. Answer: A

Explanation: Supportive listening normalizes emotions and builds trust. Transient sadness or insecurity are common during early adjustment. Empathy and education foster coping and prevent depressive escalation.
SubChapter: Emotional Support and Adaptation Counseling

Q214. Answer: A

Explanation: Fever with uterine tenderness and offensive lochia after 24 hours indicates endometritis, a uterine lining infection caused by ascending bacteria. Prompt antibiotic therapy and monitoring prevent sepsis. Mastitis involves the breast, and cystitis presents with urinary discomfort, not uterine tenderness.
SubChapter: Postpartum Infection Management

Q215. Answer: A

Explanation: Fiber and adequate fluids soften stools and stimulate bowel motility, preventing straining that could disrupt sutures or hemorrhoids. Reduced mobility and dehydration increase constipation risk, so early ambulation and balanced nutrition are encouraged for optimal gastrointestinal recovery.
SubChapter: Gastrointestinal Health Promotion

Q216. Answer: D

Explanation: A boggy, high uterus indicates subinvolution or atony causing delayed hemorrhage. Immediate fundal massage stimulates contraction and decreases bleeding. If tone does not improve, the nurse notifies the provider for possible uterotonic therapy. Documentation alone delays intervention.
SubChapter: Uterine Tone and Hemorrhage Response

Q217. Answer: A

Explanation: Dysuria and urgency indicate possible urinary tract infection. A urine culture identifies pathogens for targeted antibiotic therapy. Ice packs relieve perineal trauma but not infection. Early identification prevents ascending infection and systemic illness.
SubChapter: Urinary System Assessment

Q218. Answer: A

Explanation: Mastitis management includes continued milk removal, warm compresses, and antibiotics. Stopping feeds worsens engorgement and infection risk. Early treatment ensures milk supply maintenance and rapid recovery while preventing abscess formation.
SubChapter: Breast Infection Management

Q219. Answer: A

Explanation: Eye contact, smiling, and affectionate speech indicate positive bonding and emotional connection. Avoidance or disinterest suggests delayed attachment or postpartum mood disturbance requiring supportive intervention. Early recognition promotes healthy family adaptation and caregiving confidence.
SubChapter: Maternal–Infant Bonding Assessment

Q220. Answer: D

Explanation: Lochia normally transitions from rubra to serosa to alba by day 10, marking endometrial repair. Persistent bright bleeding or foul odor would indicate pathology. Clear understanding reassures the patient and prevents unnecessary anxiety.

SubChapter: Lochial Progression Monitoring

Q221. Answer: A

Explanation: Firm uterus with continued bleeding indicates trauma rather than atony. Cervical or vaginal tears cause brisk bleeding despite adequate tone. Prompt provider notification ensures repair and bleeding control.

SubChapter: Postpartum Hemorrhage Etiology

Q222. Answer: A

Explanation: Prolonged depression and anhedonia beyond two weeks require assessment for clinical depression. Early referral prevents deterioration and supports family well-being. Rest alone does not resolve pathologic mood disorders.

SubChapter: Mental Health and Emotional Screening

Q223. Answer: A

Explanation: Wiping front to back prevents fecal contamination of the vaginal area, reducing infection risk. Tampons and powders promote bacterial growth. Regular gentle cleansing with warm water supports healing and comfort.

SubChapter: Perineal Hygiene and Infection Prevention

Q224. Answer: C

Explanation: Sudden heavy bleeding and clots after initial improvement suggest late postpartum hemorrhage or retained tissue. Prompt evaluation ensures timely management and prevents hypovolemia or infection.

SubChapter: Delayed Hemorrhage Recognition

Q225. Answer: A

Explanation: Prolactin suppresses ovulation during exclusive breastfeeding, delaying menstruation for several months. Timing varies, and contraception is advised as ovulation may precede menses. This physiologic delay protects maternal recovery and energy balance.

SubChapter: Lactation and Reproductive Physiology

Q226. Answer: A

Explanation: Supportive communication encourages expression of fear or detachment, aiding emotional assessment. Forcing interaction or ignoring signs can worsen anxiety or depression. Empathetic support fosters confidence and attachment.

SubChapter: Emotional Adjustment and Bonding Support

Q227. Answer: A

Explanation: Intercourse is safe when perineal tissues heal and bleeding ceases, preventing infection and discomfort. Healing typically occurs by six weeks. Contraception remains necessary even while breastfeeding due to unpredictable ovulation.

SubChapter: Sexual Health and Contraception Education

Q228. Answer: D

Explanation: Fever and malodorous lochia suggest uterine infection requiring prompt medical care. Breast engorgement and mild fatigue are expected physiologic responses. Accurate teaching supports early detection and timely intervention.

SubChapter: Postpartum Infection Surveillance

Q229. Answer: A

Explanation: The uterus descends approximately one centimeter per day; by the second day it should be two centimeters below the umbilicus. Higher levels indicate subinvolution or bladder distention needing correction.

SubChapter: Uterine Involution Assessment

Q230. Answer: A

Explanation: Frequent feeding and warmth soften tissue and promote milk flow. Fluid restriction or binding worsens engorgement and increases mastitis risk. Regular emptying maintains supply and comfort.
SubChapter: Engorgement Relief and Lactation Support
Q231. Answer: A
Explanation: Localized leg pain and swelling suggest possible deep vein thrombosis, requiring urgent evaluation. Massage or ambulation risks embolus dislodgement. Early detection prevents life-threatening pulmonary embolism.
SubChapter: Circulatory Complication Management
Q232. Answer: D
Explanation: Postpartum diuresis eliminates excess extracellular fluid accumulated during pregnancy. Increased output is expected within 24–48 hours and helps prevent edema. Infection would present with pain or urgency.
SubChapter: Fluid and Renal Adaptation
Q233. Answer: A
Explanation: Purulent drainage and warmth indicate surgical wound infection requiring prompt medical evaluation and antibiotic therapy. Covering without treatment risks sepsis. Early recognition promotes healing and prevents systemic spread.
SubChapter: Surgical Site Infection Management
Q234. Answer: A
Explanation: A tense, localized swelling with disproportionate pain despite firm fundus indicates a hematoma from vessel rupture. Prompt evaluation and possible surgical drainage relieve pressure and prevent blood loss or tissue necrosis. Atony presents with uterine softness, not localized swelling.
SubChapter: Perineal Trauma Recognition
Q235. Answer: A
Explanation: Limiting heavy lifting for about six weeks protects abdominal muscles and incision integrity. Driving and bathing are postponed until cleared by the provider. Gradual mobility and wound care promote safe healing and prevent dehiscence.
SubChapter: Cesarean Postoperative Self-Care
Q236. Answer: C
Explanation: Postpartum bradycardia results from decreased cardiac workload and increased stroke volume after birth. It is physiologic if asymptomatic. Continuous observation ensures stability. Intervention is unnecessary unless accompanied by hypotension or dizziness.
SubChapter: Cardiovascular Physiologic Adaptation
Q237. Answer: A
Explanation: Proper latch covering the areola distributes pressure evenly and prevents tissue trauma. Alcohol dries skin and promotes cracking. Frequent, unrestricted feeding maintains comfort and effective milk transfer.
SubChapter: Breastfeeding Technique Instruction
Q238. Answer: A
Explanation: Bladder distention displaces the uterus laterally, causing discomfort and incomplete contraction. Encouraging urination restores uterine position and reduces pain. Fundal massage without emptying is ineffective.
SubChapter: Bladder Elimination and Uterine Position
Q239. Answer: A
Explanation: Verbalizing adaptation and confidence reflects positive transition into motherhood. Avoidance or regret suggests possible depression or bonding difficulty. Supportive follow-up reinforces coping and family adjustment.

SubChapter: Psychologic Adaptation and Coping

Q240. Answer: C

Explanation: Calcium in milk impairs iron absorption. Taking supplements with vitamin C enhances uptake, while dark stools are harmless. Prolonged use restores hemoglobin after pregnancy-related blood loss.

SubChapter: Nutritional Supplement Education

Q241. Answer: A

Explanation: Early movement and gentle leg exercises improve venous return, reducing clot formation. Immobility and dehydration increase risk. Adequate hydration and circulation maintenance are key postoperative goals.

SubChapter: Thromboembolism Prevention

Q242. Answer: A

Explanation: Warm water cleansing promotes comfort and prevents bacterial growth. Powders and tampons increase infection risk. Hygiene and dryness enhance healing and pain relief while maintaining tissue integrity.

SubChapter: Perineal Care and Infection Prevention

Q243. Answer: A

Explanation: Acknowledging anxiety normalizes the experience and allows guided teaching on safe infant handling. Supportive reassurance strengthens confidence and reduces intrusive thoughts. Ignoring concerns undermines trust and recovery.

SubChapter: Emotional Support and Parental Education

Q244. Answer: C

Explanation: Urinary burning often results from perineal wound contact with urine or infection. Inspection identifies redness or edema requiring care adjustments. Prompt management ensures comfort and prevents ascending infection.

SubChapter: Perineal Assessment and Pain Management

Q245. Answer: A

Explanation: Return to bright-red bleeding indicates subinvolution or retained tissue and risk for hemorrhage. Other signs are normal postpartum changes. Timely assessment prevents severe complications.

SubChapter: Abnormal Lochial Pattern Recognition

Q246. Answer: A

Explanation: Thrush requires concurrent antifungal therapy for mother and baby to prevent reinfection. Breastfeeding may continue with hygiene measures. Alcohol damages tissue; milk remains safe if handled properly.

SubChapter: Lactation Infection Management

Q247. Answer: A

Explanation: Joyful interaction and self-efficacy signal successful maternal adaptation. Withdrawal, overexertion, or persistent sadness suggest maladjustment or depression requiring evaluation. Emotional support strengthens parental competence.

SubChapter: Maternal Role Adaptation

Q248. Answer: D

Explanation: Fever and localized swelling indicate wound infection or abscess formation. Prompt reporting ensures culture and antibiotic therapy, preventing systemic spread. Tight dressings or ignoring signs delay treatment.

SubChapter: Post-Cesarean Infection Recognition

Q249. Answer: A

Explanation: Regular feeding and hydration stimulate milk production via oxytocin and prolactin release. Skipping feeds decreases supply; nutrition supports sustained energy and milk quality.
SubChapter: Lactation Maintenance Counseling

Q250. Answer: A

Explanation: Emotional instability persisting beyond two weeks, accompanied by anxiety or concentration issues, indicates postpartum depression needing assessment and therapy. Normal fatigue resolves with rest; infection presents with fever, not mood changes.
SubChapter: Psychological Health Assessment

Q251. Answer: A

Explanation: Warm sitz baths enhance circulation, reduce pain, and promote venous drainage. Continuous ice beyond early period decreases comfort. Adequate fluids and diet prevent recurrence.
SubChapter: Perineal Comfort and Self-Care

Q252. Answer: D

Explanation: The uterus should descend approximately 1 cm per day; by day 5 it lies midway and firm. Boggy or deviated findings suggest atony or bladder distention needing correction.
SubChapter: Uterine Involution Monitoring

Q253. Answer: A

Explanation: Active listening and emotional validation support psychological recovery and help integrate the birth experience. Suppression or dismissal impedes adjustment and trust. Compassionate communication enhances coping and bonding.
SubChapter: Therapeutic Communication and Emotional Support

Chapter 3

Q254. Answer: A

Explanation: Nasal flaring signals increased respiratory effort from airway obstruction or distress, warranting prompt support. Irregular respirations during sleep are normal transitional findings. Occasional sneezing helps clear nasal passages, not distress. Brief acrocyanosis reflects normal peripheral perfusion adjustment after birth, not hypoxia.
SubChapter: Respiratory Adaptation

Q255. Answer: A

Explanation: A heart rate of 85 bpm often improves with gentle stimulation due to transient vagal response or sleep state. Chest compressions are reserved for rates below 60 bpm. Resuscitation activation is premature here. Environmental temperature changes have little immediate cardiac effect.
SubChapter: Cardiovascular Assessment

Q256. Answer: C

Explanation: Absent femoral pulses may indicate coarctation of the aorta, a critical congenital defect needing prompt evaluation. Molding and suture overlap are normal birth findings. Mild temperature variation is expected as thermoregulation stabilizes post-delivery.
SubChapter: Cardiovascular Assessment

Q257. Answer: B

Explanation: Feeding corrects mild asymptomatic hypoglycemia (30–45 mg/dL) by promoting glucose utilization and thermogenesis. IV dextrose is indicated for severe or symptomatic cases. Delaying recheck or notifying before intervention can risk neuroglycopenia.
SubChapter: Metabolic Adaptation

Q258. Answer: B

Explanation: Periodic breathing under 10 seconds without color change is normal in newborns due to immature respiratory control. Rates below 30 are bradypneic, grunting and retractions indicate distress requiring evaluation.
SubChapter: Respiratory Assessment

Q259. Answer: D

Explanation: A single umbilical artery may indicate renal or cardiac anomalies; further imaging is required. Routine care and cleaning are standard but insufficient evaluation. Antibiotic ointment is unnecessary unless infection signs occur.

SubChapter: Physical Assessment

Q260. Answer: B

Explanation: The Babinski reflex—toe dorsiflexion with fanning—is normal until 12–18 months, signifying intact corticospinal tracts. Absent rooting or dilated pupils suggest neurologic issues; jaundice spreading to the legs signals pathologic hyperbilirubinemia.

SubChapter: Neurologic Assessment

Q261. Answer: B

Explanation: Hypoglycemia commonly causes neonatal jitteriness; glucose check confirms etiology. Hypocalcemia may also contribute but is secondary consideration. Temperature or bilirubin changes produce different symptom patterns, not neuromuscular tremors.

SubChapter: Metabolic Assessment

Q262. Answer: D

Explanation: Eye and mouth exams may distress infants; conducting them last maintains calm for accurate baseline vitals. Cardiopulmonary and abdominal exams are best while quiet. Genital inspection causes minimal disturbance.

SubChapter: Physical Examination Technique

Q263. Answer: B

Explanation: Hypothermia below 36°C requires active rewarming to prevent metabolic acidosis and hypoglycemia. Observation or feeding alone cannot reverse thermal loss. Sepsis workup follows if temperature fails to stabilize after warming.

SubChapter: Thermoregulation

Q264. Answer: B

Explanation: Ductus arteriosus closure marks successful circulatory adaptation to air breathing. Persistent or central cyanosis suggests hypoxemia or cardiac defects. Murmur plus weak pulses indicates obstructive pathology, not normal transition.

SubChapter: Cardiovascular Transition

Q265. Answer: C

Explanation: Sustained tachycardia over 180 bpm indicates distress, dehydration, or infection. Respiratory sinus arrhythmia and mild murmurs are transient findings. Early acrocyanosis reflects immature peripheral circulation, typically resolving within hours.

SubChapter: Cardiovascular Assessment

Q266. Answer: B

Explanation: Skin-to-skin contact conserves heat via conduction and reduces cold stress. Immediate drying minimizes evaporative loss. Bathing or cooling causes hypothermia, while delayed drying increases thermal instability and energy expenditure.

SubChapter: Thermoregulation

Q267. Answer: A

Explanation: Grunting and retractions reflect alveolar collapse and inadequate surfactant—classic of RDS. Periodic breathing and acrocyanosis are benign. Sneezing or hiccups indicate normal reflex activity, not pulmonary compromise.

SubChapter: Respiratory Compromise

Q268. Answer: B

Explanation: Hematoma breakdown increases bilirubin load, predisposing to jaundice. Glucose, calcium, and temperature changes are unrelated unless systemic instability develops.

SubChapter: Hematologic Adaptation

Q269. Answer: C

Explanation: The rooting reflex enables infants to turn toward nipple stimulation, aiding effective feeding. Moro tests neurologic integrity; palmar and stepping are developmental motor reflexes unrelated to nutrition.

SubChapter: Neurologic Reflexes

Q270. Answer: C

Explanation: Moderate lanugo and vernix signify typical term maturity. Excess lanugo suggests prematurity; absence indicates postmaturity. These are normal protective findings, not pathologic.

SubChapter: Physical Characteristics

Q271. Answer: C

Explanation: Facial grimacing, especially brow bulge and crying, strongly correlate with physiologic pain responses. Yawning, sucking, or rooting are self-soothing or feeding behaviors, not pain indicators.

SubChapter: Pain Assessment

Q272. Answer: A

Explanation: Caput succedaneum is serosanguinous edema crossing sutures due to birth pressure. Cephalohematoma (under periosteum) does not cross lines. Bruising or hemorrhage are distinct, often deeper injuries requiring monitoring.

SubChapter: Birth Trauma Assessment

Q273. Answer: B

Explanation: Current NRP guidelines advise airway clearing only if secretions obstruct breathing to prevent vagal stimulation. Routine suctioning may cause bradycardia. Drying precedes feeding to conserve heat and energy.

SubChapter: Immediate Newborn Care

Q274. Answer: B

Explanation: Airway patency ensures oxygenation and survival, the highest newborn priority. Reflexes and skin findings are secondary once breathing is effective. Cord color has limited initial importance unless signs of infection exist.

SubChapter: Immediate Stabilization

Q275. Answer: A

Explanation: Transient tachypnea arises from delayed lung fluid clearance, common in term cesarean births. It resolves within 24–48 hours. Persistent hypertension or aspiration produce severe hypoxia; RDS is more typical of prematurity.

SubChapter: Respiratory Adaptation

Q276. Answer: B

Explanation: Temperature instability (hypo or hyperthermia) frequently signals sepsis because neonates lack immune thermoregulation. Mild jaundice and acrocyanosis are expected transitions; pink mucosa suggests adequate oxygenation.

SubChapter: Infection Assessment

Q277. Answer: A

Explanation: Physiologic splitting of S2 occurs with respiratory pressure changes and closes spontaneously within days. Continuous or fixed sounds imply congenital defects like PDA or ASD. Harsh murmurs warrant evaluation.

SubChapter: Cardiac Auscultation

Q278. Answer: C

Explanation: Combined weight, length, and head circumference enable gestational age classification and growth curve placement. Single measures can mislead due to fluid loss or cranial molding. Chest circumference adds limited value for routine screening.

SubChapter: Growth Assessment

Q279. Answer: B

Explanation: Hematocrit > 65 % indicates polycythemia causing sluggish circulation and hypoglycemia risk. Anemia is opposite; bleeding and infection are unrelated unless complicated. Early hydration and monitoring prevent thrombotic events.

SubChapter: Hematologic Assessment

Q280. Answer: B

Explanation: Evaporative loss occurs from amniotic fluid on skin; prompt drying minimizes cooling. Room warmth reduces radiation, not evaporation. Delayed capping or metal avoidance address conduction loss, less immediate than drying.

SubChapter: Thermal Management

Q281. Answer: A

Explanation: Mild hypothermia requires controlled rewarming to prevent metabolic stress and hypoglycemia. Glucose gel is secondary if symptoms persist. Antibiotics or delay are inappropriate without infection evidence.

SubChapter: Thermoregulation

Q282. Answer: B

Explanation: Erythema toxicum appears as blotchy macules and resolves spontaneously; it is a normal immunologic reaction. Petechiae or cyanosis suggest pathology, while early jaundice signals hemolysis or infection.

SubChapter: Dermatologic Findings

Q283. Answer: B

Explanation: Stepping reflex fades around 2 months as weight increases and motor control develops. Moro and grasp persist to 4 months; rooting lasts until feeding matures. Premature loss suggests neurologic abnormality.

SubChapter: Neuromuscular Assessment

Q284. Answer: C

Explanation: Infants of diabetic mothers experience rebound hypoglycemia from maternal hyperinsulinemia exposure. Preterm or postterm status can increase risk but less predictably. Term AGA infants maintain stable glucose better.

SubChapter: Metabolic Monitoring

Q285. Answer: C

Explanation: Bilious vomiting and distention imply intestinal obstruction such as malrotation. Pyloric stenosis causes non-bilious projectile emesis. Reflux or NEC present later with feeding intolerance or bloody stool.

SubChapter: Gastrointestinal Assessment

Q286. Answer: A

Explanation: Scaphoid abdomen plus respiratory distress suggests diaphragmatic hernia with abdominal contents in thorax. Other findings are normal transitional states. Immediate airway management is vital.

SubChapter: Abdominal Assessment

Q287. Answer: C

Explanation: Adequate hydration produces ≥6 wet diapers by day 3–4, confirming milk intake. Lower counts indicate dehydration or feeding issues. Output does not remain variable beyond the first few days.

SubChapter: Fluid Balance

Q288. Answer: B

Explanation: Bilirubin of 10 mg/dL at 24 hours suggests physiologic rise but requires hydration and repeat testing. Phototherapy threshold is usually ≥12–15 mg/dL. Stopping breastfeeding is contraindicated unless pathologic jaundice confirmed.
SubChapter: Hepatic Assessment
Q289. Answer: B
Explanation: Normal oxygenation produces rosy color and saturation > 95 %. Central cyanosis or SpO_2 below 90 % imply hypoxemia. Peripheral cyanosis alone is acceptable in early transition.
SubChapter: Respiratory Monitoring
Q290. Answer: A
Explanation: Grunting and flaring indicate respiratory distress requiring oxygen support and evaluation. Feeding increases oxygen demand; swaddling delays care and risk decompensation. Prompt response prevents hypoxemia.
SubChapter: Respiratory Distress Response
Q291. Answer: A
Explanation: Hypocalcemia manifests as neuromuscular irritability with tremors and shrill cry. Lethargy fits hypoglycemia; flushed skin or bradycardia stem from other causes. Early identification prevents seizures.
SubChapter: Electrolyte Assessment
Q292. Answer: A
Explanation: Persistent murmurs beyond 48 hours may signal cardiac anomalies needing echocardiography. Epstein pearls and erythema toxicum are benign; acrocyanosis resolves spontaneously.
SubChapter: Cardiac Follow-Up
Q293. Answer: C
Explanation: Failed initial hearing screens require retesting within 2 weeks and parent education per EHDI guidelines. Immediate retesting post-feeding is ineffective due to residual fluid. Antibiotics are not indicated without infection.
SubChapter: Sensory Assessment
Q294. Answer: A
Explanation: Capillary refill < 3 seconds indicates stable cardiac output and tissue perfusion. Prolonged acrocyanosis or cool limbs signal poor flow. Systolic < 50 mm Hg in term infants is abnormally low and may indicate shock.
SubChapter: Circulatory Assessment
Q295. Answer: B
Explanation: Respiratory rates 30–60 breaths/min with clear lungs are normal for newborns. Oxygen or feeding delay is unnecessary. Notification is reserved for tachypnea or distress signs like retractions.
SubChapter: Respiratory Assessment
Q296. Answer: A
Explanation: Hypothermic newborns show lethargy and bradycardia from metabolic slowdown. Infection commonly produces tachypnea and poor feeding with temperature instability. Apnea and pallor represent severe decompensation, not specific to hypothermia.
SubChapter: Thermoregulatory Assessment
Q297. Answer: A
Explanation: Soft intermittent murmurs with crying are often transitional from flow turbulence as ductus closes. Constant or loud murmurs may signal structural defects like VSD or stenosis.
SubChapter: Cardiac Assessment
Q298. Answer: A

Explanation: Active cry and movements signify vigorous neurologic function and oxygenation. Distention, retractions, or cyanosis suggest distress requiring evaluation.
SubChapter: Neurologic and Vital Signs Assessment

Q299. Answer: A

Explanation: Up to 10 % weight loss is normal as fluid balance adjusts; frequent feeding prevents excess loss. IV or supplement intervention is reserved for > 10 % loss or clinical dehydration.
SubChapter: Fluid and Nutrition Assessment

Q300. Answer: B

Explanation: Flexion and active movement demonstrate normal tone and neurologic integrity. Limpness, asymmetry, or weak suck suggest injury or immaturity.
SubChapter: Neuromotor Assessment

Questions (301-400)

Q301. A preterm infant shows flaring and grunting at 2 hours old. What is the nurse's priority?

A. Assess oxygen saturation and apply CPAP
B. Begin oral feeding
C. Place in side-lying position only
D. Observe without intervention

Q302. Which sign indicates pathologic jaundice?

A. Appears within first 24 hours of life
B. Begins after day 2 and resolves by day 5
C. Total bilirubin below 12 mg/dL at 48 hours
D. Occurs in breastfed infants only

Q303. Which parameter best indicates adequate hydration in newborns?

A. Moist mucous membranes and tears
B. Weight loss > 10 %
C. Sunken fontanelles
D. Dry lips and urine crystals

Q304. A newborn with tachypnea has SpO_2 92 %. Which action is appropriate?

A. Place under radiant warmer and reassess
B. Initiate supplemental oxygen per protocol
C. Feed to calm infant
D. Ignore if no retractions

Q305. Which assessment best evaluates neurologic maturity?

A. Rooting reflex
B. Heel-to-ear maneuver and square window test
C. Skin texture and vernix amount
D. Presence of lanugo

Q306. Which sign indicates adequate pain management after heel stick?

A. Stable heart rate and quiet alert state
B. Persistent crying for 10 minutes
C. Flaccid posture and pallor
D. Rapid breathing and grimacing

Q307. Which finding is normal in a term newborn's abdomen?

A. Palpable liver 1–2 cm below costal margin
B. Distended, tense abdomen
C. Absent bowel sounds
D. Visible veins over abdominal wall

Q308. The nurse notes a newborn's glucose is 28 mg/dL with tremors. Next action?

A. Administer IV dextrose per protocol
B. Feed and recheck in 1 hour
C. Continue observation
D. Delay intervention until symptoms progress

Q309. Which finding in a term infant requires reporting?

A. Fontanelle pulsating with crying
B. Flat fontanelle when upright
C. Anterior fontanelle bulging at rest
D. Posterior fontanelle closed by 2 months

Q310. Which physical finding suggests post-term gestation?

A. Peeling skin and long fingernails
B. Abundant vernix and lanugo
C. Flat areolae with no breast tissue
D. Soft ear cartilage

Q311. A newborn's hematocrit is 58 %. What does this mean?
A. Normal value for term infant
B. Anemic condition
C. Need for exchange transfusion
D. Possible hemorrhage

Q312. Which intervention best reduces pain during heel puncture?
A. Oral sucrose before procedure
B. Pacifier after procedure
C. Applying ice before puncture
D. Delaying feeding for accuracy

Q313. Which observation requires immediate intervention during newborn assessment?
A. Startle response after noise
B. Periodic breathing with no cyanosis
C. Apnea lasting 15 seconds with color change
D. Transient tremors after crying

Q314. Which newborn finding is a sign of respiratory distress?
A. Irregular respirations without color change
B. Nasal flaring with grunting
C. Quiet breathing during sleep
D. Brief apnea < 10 seconds

Q315. A newborn's temperature is 95 °F (35 °C) after delivery. Which nursing action is priority?
A. Place skin-to-skin with mother and cover with warm blanket
B. Feed the infant immediately
C. Delay warming to avoid shock
D. Begin oxygen therapy

Q316. A neonate has a blood glucose of 28 mg/dL but is asymptomatic. What should the nurse do?
A. Feed immediately and recheck in 30 minutes
B. Begin IV dextrose
C. Observe and retest in 6 hours
D. Notify physician without intervention

Q317. Which assessment finding suggests early sepsis in a newborn?
A. Pink skin and active crying
B. Poor feeding and temperature instability
C. Mild acrocyanosis
D. Transient tachypnea after birth

Q318. Which finding indicates the need for further neurologic evaluation?
A. Tremors after crying
B. Absence of Moro reflex
C. Rooting and sucking reflexes present
D. Symmetric movement of limbs

Q319. The nurse notes delayed urine output 24 hours after birth. What should be done first?
A. Assess hydration and intake
B. Insert a urinary catheter
C. Administer IV fluids

D. Notify provider immediately for renal failure

Q320. Which finding requires follow-up before discharge?

A. Weight loss of 9 %
B. Umbilical cord dry and separating
C. Heart murmur persistent beyond 48 hours
D. Slight peeling skin

Q321. Which action best supports the neonate's immune protection?

A. Delay first feeding 24 hours
B. Encourage early breastfeeding
C. Bathe immediately after birth
D. Isolate infant from mother

Q322. Which skin finding is pathologic in a newborn?

A. Mongolian spot
B. Petechiae over trunk and face
C. Erythema toxicum
D. Milia on nose

Q323. Which vital sign pattern is typical for a healthy term newborn?

A. HR 160 bpm, RR 50, Temp 98.6 °F
B. HR 90 bpm, RR 25, Temp 96 °F
C. HR 190 bpm, RR 70, Temp 99.5 °F
D. HR 110 bpm, RR 30, Temp 100.5 °F

Q324. Which finding indicates adequate respiratory transition?

A. SpO_2 97 % on room air after 10 minutes
B. Cyanosis of lips at 20 minutes
C. Apnea for 20 seconds
D. RR 80 with grunting

Q325. A newborn presents with a large anterior fontanelle and wide sutures. What should the nurse suspect?

A. Normal variant
B. Hypothyroidism or increased ICP
C. Dehydration
D. Premature closure

Q326. A nurse observes an umbilical cord with one artery and one vein. Next step?

A. Document as normal variant
B. Request renal ultrasound evaluation
C. Clamp cord again
D. Cleanse with alcohol daily

Q327. Which finding indicates adequate thermoregulation after birth?

A. Pink skin, axillary temp 98.2 °F
B. Cool extremities, temp 96.5 °F
C. Shivering response
D. Apnea with temperature drop

Q328. Which assessment is critical before discharge to detect critical congenital heart disease (CCHD)?

A. Pulse oximetry screening on hand and foot
B. Auscultate heart sounds only
C. Palpate femoral pulses once
D. Assess capillary refill time

Q329. Which behavior indicates effective newborn adaptation during the second period of reactivity?

A. Deep sleep state
B. Increased alertness and interest in feeding
C. Reduced muscle tone and lethargy
D. Hypothermia with irregular breathing

Q330. Which assessment is priority after circumcision?
A. Observe for bleeding and urination
B. Apply tight pressure dressing
C. Clean with alcohol swabs
D. Bathe infant immediately

Q331. Which finding during eye assessment is normal in newborns?
A. Intermittent strabismus
B. Purulent discharge
C. Cloudy cornea
D. Absence of red reflex

Q332. The nurse notes a cephalohematoma. What is the primary complication to monitor?
A. Hyperbilirubinemia
B. Infection of scalp
C. Increased ICP
D. Cranial fracture

Q333. A term infant displays hands and feet cyanotic with pink trunk at 10 minutes. What is the appropriate response?
A. Perform pulse oximetry and admit to NICU
B. Administer oxygen via mask
C. Call provider for cyanosis
D. Continue to monitor; normal acrocyanosis

Q334. Which finding is considered abnormal in a newborn's musculoskeletal assessment?
A. Equal leg lengths and symmetric gluteal folds
B. Limited hip abduction with clicking sound
C. Flexed arms and legs at rest
D. Strong grasp reflex

Q335. Which behavior best indicates effective thermoregulation?
A. Quiet alert state and pink skin tone
B. Jitteriness and irritability
C. Peripheral cyanosis and hypoglycemia
D. Weak cry and cool extremities

Q336. A newborn's abdomen appears distended and firm. What is the nurse's next step?
A. Assess for bowel sounds and passage of meconium
B. Feed to relieve gas
C. Document as normal finding
D. Massage abdomen gently

Q337. The nurse observes jitteriness and poor feeding in a newborn. Which lab should be checked first?
A. Serum bilirubin
B. Blood glucose
C. Hemoglobin
D. Calcium level

Q338时光. Which assessment indicates abnormal neurologic function in a newborn?

A. Symmetric Moro reflex
B. Weak or absent suck reflex
C. Rooting reflex present
D. Flexed extremities

Q339. Which physical finding is typical in a postterm infant?
A. Cracked, peeling skin
B. Abundant vernix
C. Lanugo covering shoulders
D. Soft ear cartilage

Q340. The nurse notes intermittent stridor in a neonate. What is the likely cause?
A. Laryngomalacia
B. Choanal atresia
C. Diaphragmatic hernia
D. Pneumothorax

Q341. Which finding requires provider notification in a term infant?
A. Umbilical stump moist but without redness
B. Temperature of 97.9 °F
C. Respiratory rate of 75 with grunting
D. Irregular heart rate during sleep

Q342. The nurse observes generalized jaundice at 12 hours old. What action is priority?
A. Obtain a bilirubin level immediately
B. Encourage frequent breastfeeding only
C. Observe for 24 hours
D. Provide sunlight exposure

Q343. Which nursing action reduces risk of cold stress in a newborn during bathing?
A. Warm the water and limit bath duration
B. Keep the newborn wet to retain vernix
C. Use air drying technique
D. Bathe immediately after birth

Q344. What finding suggests adequate fluid intake in a breastfeeding infant?
A. Six or more wet diapers per day after day 4
B. Weight loss > 10 %
C. No stool for 24 hours
D. Dry mucous membranes

Q345. Which newborn requires further cardiac evaluation?
A. Capillary refill under 2 seconds
B. Pink color with acrocyanosis
C. Transient murmur that disappears after 12 hours
D. SpO_2 89 % at 10 minutes on room air

Q346. Which sign is most consistent with neonatal pain?
A. Brow bulge and high-pitched cry
B. Regular respirations and relaxed posture
C. Steady heart rate
D. Sleep between feedings

Q347. A newborn's abdomen shows visible bowel loops and scaphoid appearance. What condition is suspected?
A. Congenital diaphragmatic hernia
B. Necrotizing enterocolitis

C. Pyloric stenosis
D. Omphalocele

Q348. Which action ensures accuracy during newborn temperature measurement?
A. Use axillary site with digital thermometer
B. Rectal measurement for all infants
C. Oral measurement if infant is quiet
D. Tympanic thermometer within 1 hour of birth

Q349. Which finding at birth suggests intrauterine growth restriction (IUGR)?
A. Strong subcutaneous fat folds
B. Large body with abundant fat
C. Vernix and lanugo covering trunk
D. Loose, dry skin and wide anterior fontanelle

Q350. Which reflex assists the newborn with protection during sudden movements?
A. Moro reflex
B. Rooting reflex
C. Babinski reflex
D. Stepping reflex

Q351. Which assessment finding indicates normal adaptation in newborn circulation?
A. Closure of foramen ovale
B. Persistent ductus arteriosus
C. Weak femoral pulses
D. Central cyanosis

Q352. Which newborn is at greatest risk for hypothermia?
A. Preterm infant with minimal brown fat
B. Term infant skin-to-skin after birth
C. Large-for-gestational-age infant
D. Infant dressed and swaddled

Q353. A newborn's glucose remains < 40 mg/dL despite feeding. What is the next nursing action?
A. Keep infant under warmer only
B. Reattempt feeding in 4 hours
C. Start IV dextrose infusion
D. Notify mother to increase feeding frequency

Q354. A newborn's Apgar score at 1 minute is 4. What is the nurse's priority?
A. Begin positive pressure ventilation
B. Start chest compressions
C. Assess temperature
D. Administer glucose

Q355. Which characteristic is normal in a healthy term newborn's skin?
A. Vernix in body creases
B. Generalized cyanosis
C. Yellow tint at 8 hours
D. Petechiae over trunk

Q356. What does a high-pitched cry in a newborn suggest?
A. Neurologic disturbance or withdrawal
B. Normal hunger response
C. Mild respiratory congestion
D. Overstimulation

Q357. A nurse palpates a soft, flat anterior fontanelle in a quiet newborn. How should this be interpreted?

A. Late anemia

B. Early dehydration

C. Increased intracranial pressure

D. Normal finding

Q358. Which newborn finding warrants immediate evaluation?

A. Asymmetrical movement of arms during Moro reflex

B. Jitteriness after crying

C. Acrocyanosis at 15 minutes

D. Irregular respirations while sleeping

Q359. A term newborn's hematocrit is 70%. What complication should the nurse monitor for?

A. Hypoglycemia and hyperviscosity

B. Hypocalcemia

C. Anemia

D. Sepsis

Q360. Which finding in a newborn's mouth requires further evaluation?

A. White plaques on tongue that cannot be wiped off

B. Epstein pearls on the hard palate

C. Moist pink mucosa

D. Strong suck reflex

Q361. Which finding indicates adequate renal adaptation?

A. Bloody urine

B. No void within 24 hours

C. Dark amber urine with crystals

D. Urine output of 1–3 mL/kg/hr

Q362. What does a ruddy complexion in a newborn suggest?

A. Polycythemia

B. Anemia

C. Hypothermia

D. Hypoxia

Q363. Which step should the nurse take before performing a newborn heel stick?

A. Warm the heel for 3–5 minutes

B. Clean with alcohol and puncture deeply

C. Choose the arch of the foot

D. Use the same site for repeat sampling

Q364. A newborn exhibits mild tremors when disturbed but normal tone and feeding. Interpretation?

A. Normal newborn behavior

B. Hypocalcemia

C. Hypoglycemia

D. Sepsis

Q365. A 1-day-old infant has RR 65, HR 140, mild nasal flaring. What is the nurse's next action?

A. Delay feeding

B. Initiate oxygen therapy

C. Prepare for intubation

D. Monitor and reassess in 1 hour

Q366. Which assessment should be completed before a newborn is discharged?

A. Hearing screen and critical congenital heart disease screening

B. Vitamin K administration
C. Hepatitis B vaccine
D. Umbilical cord care teaching

Q367. Which newborn finding suggests respiratory distress syndrome (RDS)?
A. Grunting, retractions, cyanosis
B. Transient tachypnea
C. Mild nasal flaring resolving after 30 minutes
D. Respirations 40/min, no retractions

Q368. Which nursing intervention minimizes evaporative heat loss?
A. Drying the infant immediately after birth
B. Using warm blankets over the warmer
C. Avoiding metal surfaces
D. Covering head after 2 hours

Q369. What is the likely cause of a newborn's blood glucose of 33 mg/dL with jitteriness?
A. HypercalcemiaV
B. Excess bilirubin breakdown
C. Inadequate glycogen stores or delayed feeding
D. Cold stress

Q370. A nurse notices asymmetric chest movement after delivery. What should be suspected?
A. Pneumothorax or fractured clavicle
B. Normal transitional breathing
C. Upper airway obstruction
D. Diaphragmatic hernia

Q371. Which assessment best evaluates peripheral circulation in a newborn?
A. Capillary refill time
B. Heart rate alone
C. Skin temperature
D. Blood pressure reading

Q372. Which finding is consistent with a normal transitional period?
A. Irregular respirations without cyanosis
B. Grunting and severe retractions
C. Pale skin and lethargy
D. Temperature 35 °C (95 °F)

Q373. Which finding would the nurse expect in an infant with mild hypothermia?
A. Bradycardia and high temperature
B. Decreased respiratory rate and hyperglycemia
C. Increased oxygen consumption and hypoglycemia
D. Seizure activity

Q374. A nurse notices nasal flaring and intercostal retractions in a newborn. What does this indicate?
A. Respiratory distress
B. Normal periodic breathing
C. Overstimulation
D. Nasal congestion

Q375. Which newborn is at greatest risk for hypoglycemia?
A. Infant of a diabetic mother
B. Term infant small for gestational age
C. Postterm infant with normal weight
D. Preterm infant with adequate weight

Q376. What finding indicates adequate hydration in a 4-day-old infant?
A. Six or more wet diapers per day
B. Sunken fontanelle
C. Dry lips and concentrated urine
D. Weight loss 12% below birth weight
Q377. A newborn's temperature drops to 95.8°F (35.4°C). Which metabolic change should the nurse anticipate?
A. Stable acid-base balance
B. Decreased metabolic rate
C. Elevated blood glucose
D. Increased glucose and oxygen consumption
Q378. Which assessment finding requires provider notification?
A. Persistent tachypnea without distress signs
B. Heart rate 100 bpm when sleeping
C. SpO_2 88% on room air
D. Soft systolic murmur first 12 hours
Q379. Which finding would the nurse expect in a term infant experiencing polycythemia?
A. Ruddy skin and lethargy
B. Pallor and tachycardia
C. Jaundice and hypothermia
D. Acrocyanosis and jitteriness
Q380. Which intervention best supports thermal stability in the immediate postpartum period?
A. Skin-to-skin contact with mother
B. Swaddling after 2 hours
C. Delay drying to preserve vernix
D. Bathing under radiant warmer
Q381. Which newborn condition requires isolation precautions?
A. Suspected neonatal herpes infection
B. Physiologic jaundice
C. Caput succedaneum
D. Cephalohematoma
Q382. A 36-hour-old newborn develops jaundice. Which interpretation is correct?
A. Biliary atresia
B. Pathologic hemolysis
C. Physiologic bilirubin rise
D. Infection-related cholestasis
Q383. Which finding is considered abnormal during newborn eye assessment?
A. Absent red reflex
B. Transient strabismus
C. Subconjunctival hemorrhage
D. Mild edema of eyelids
Q384. Which action should be performed when assessing a newborn's respiratory rate?
A. Count for a full 60 seconds
B. Count for 15 seconds and multiply by 4
C. Assess while the infant is crying
D. Perform immediately after feeding
Q385. A term newborn has mild nasal flaring and RR 70. What condition is most likely?
A. Transient tachypnea of the newborn (TTN)

B. Meconium aspiration
C. Respiratory distress syndrome
D. Pneumothorax

Q386. Which characteristic describes normal neonatal behavior?
A. Persistent irritability
B. No reaction to loud sound
C. Startles easily and then relaxes
D. Continuous sleep beyond 10 hours

Q387. A newborn's SpO_2 is 92% at 10 minutes on room air. What is the nurse's action?
A. Apply supplemental oxygen and reassess
B. Continue monitoring only
C. Delay intervention 30 minutes
D. Begin feeding to increase energy

Q388. Which finding requires urgent intervention in a term infant?
A. Apnea lasting 20 seconds with color change
B. Irregular respirations while sleeping
C. Mild tremors after feeding
D. Acrocyanosis at 15 minutes

Q389. Which physical feature is expected in a late preterm infant?
A. Smooth soles with few creases
B. Fully developed breast tissue
C. Firm ear cartilage
D. Peeling, dry skin

Q390. Which behavior indicates effective bonding?
A. Parent focuses on self-recovery only
B. Parent avoids touching infant
C. Parent maintains prolonged eye contact during feeding
D. Parent requests nurse to feed every time

Q391. Which newborn finding requires immediate evaluation for infection?
A. Temperature instability and respiratory distress
B. Mild acrocyanosis
C. Jaundice at 48 hours
D. Weight loss 8% at day 3

Q392. Which sign indicates possible hypocalcemia in a newborn?
A. Jitteriness and high-pitched cry
B. Hypothermia and bradycardia
C. Cyanosis and tachypnea
D. Poor feeding and lethargy only

Q393. What should the nurse assess first when a newborn's temperature drops?
A. Blood glucose level
B. Heart rate
C. Urine output
D. Skin color

Q394. Which newborn assessment requires immediate intervention?
A. Transient murmurs
B. Acrocyanosis of hands and feet
C. Central cyanosis of lips and tongue
D. Irregular respirations during sleep

Q395. Which sign suggests cold stress in a newborn?
A. Mottled skin and lethargy
B. Pink, warm skin
C. Regular respirations and stable temperature
D. Quiet alert state
Q396. Which newborn is at highest risk for developing respiratory distress syndrome?
A. Preterm infant born at 32 weeks
B. Term infant with meconium-stained fluid
C. Postterm infant with cracked skin
D. Small-for-gestational-age infant
Q397. What finding indicates a normal newborn cardiovascular transition?
A. Heart rate 140 bpm with strong femoral pulses
B. Persistent cyanosis after crying
C. Capillary refill > 4 seconds
D. Murmur and weak peripheral pulses
Q398. Which nursing action helps prevent conductive heat loss?
A. Using radiant warmer
B. Drying immediately after birth
C. Placing infant on a warm blanket or preheated surface
D. Covering head with hat
Q399. Which finding suggests possible congenital hypothyroidism?
A. Large fontanelle, protruding tongue, hypotonia
B. Tremors, high-pitched cry, hyperactivity
C. Pale skin and poor perfusion
D. Persistent tachypnea
Q400. What is the nurse's priority during the first 30 minutes of life?
A. Maintain airway, breathing, and temperature
B. Assess feeding reflexes
C. Perform full physical examination
D. Administer prophylactic medications

Answer key and Explanation (301-400)

Q301. Answer: A
Explanation: Flaring and grunting indicate alveolar collapse; CPAP supports functional residual capacity and improves oxygenation. Feeding and passive positioning delay critical respiratory support.
SubChapter: Respiratory Management

Q302. Answer: A
Explanation: Jaundice appearing < 24 hours suggests hemolysis or disease and requires immediate evaluation. Physiologic jaundice appears after day 2 and self-resolves. Bilirubin < 12 mg/dL is usually benign.
SubChapter: Hepatic Function

Q303. Answer: A
Explanation: Moist membranes and presence of tears reflect proper hydration. Excess weight loss or sunken fontanelle indicates dehydration. Crystals suggest concentrated urine from fluid deficit.
SubChapter: Fluid Balance

Q304. Answer: B
Explanation: Oxygen below 94 % requires support to maintain adequate tissue perfusion. Thermal or feeding actions don't address oxygen deficit. Prompt correction prevents hypoxemia.
SubChapter: Respiratory Support

Q305. Answer: B
Explanation: Heel-to-ear and square window assess flexor tone, key neurologic maturity indicators. Skin and lanugo measure physical maturity instead. Rooting tests feeding readiness, not maturity grading.
SubChapter: Neurologic Maturity

Q306. Answer: A
Explanation: Stable vitals and quiet alertness indicate comfort. Persistent crying, pallor, or grimace reflect ongoing pain requiring intervention like swaddling or sucrose.
SubChapter: Pain Assessment

Q307. Answer: A
Explanation: Slightly palpable liver is normal due to size relative to body. Distention or absent sounds indicate obstruction. Prominent veins suggest portal hypertension or ascites.
SubChapter: Abdominal Assessment

Q308. Answer: A
Explanation: Symptomatic hypoglycemia (< 30 mg/dL) requires IV dextrose to prevent neurologic injury. Feeding alone is insufficient for severe cases. Observation risks seizure and brain damage.
SubChapter: Metabolic Management

Q309. Answer: C
Explanation: Persistent bulging fontanelle indicates increased ICP or infection. Flat or pulsating with cry is normal. Posterior closure by 2 months is expected developmentally.
SubChapter: Neurologic Assessment

Q310. Answer: A
Explanation: Peeling skin and nail overgrowth indicate extended gestation with vernix loss. Other features are preterm markers reflecting immaturity.
SubChapter: Gestational Age Assessment

Q311. Answer: A
Explanation: Normal hematocrit range for term newborns is 45–65 %. Values within this are physiologic. Higher suggests polycythemia; lower reflects anemia or hemorrhage.
SubChapter: Hematologic Norms

Q312. Answer: A

Explanation: Oral sucrose activates endogenous opioid pathways, reducing pain during minor procedures. Pacifiers aid soothing but less effective alone. Ice or delayed feeding increase stress.
SubChapter: Pain Management

Q313. Answer: C

Explanation: Apnea > 15 seconds with color change suggests apneic spell requiring stimulation and evaluation for CNS or respiratory pathology. Periodic breathing or startle are normal neonatal patterns.
SubChapter: Respiratory Pathophysiology

Q314. Answer: B

Explanation: Nasal flaring and grunting indicate effort to maintain alveolar inflation and suggest distress from hypoxia or lung fluid retention. Irregular respirations and brief apnea are normal patterns in transitioning newborns and require no intervention unless accompanied by color change or bradycardia.
SubChapter: Respiratory Assessment

Q315. Answer: A

Explanation: Skin-to-skin contact is the first-line intervention for hypothermia, promoting conduction heat transfer and stabilizing vitals. Feeding and oxygen do not correct temperature loss directly, and delaying warming risks metabolic acidosis and hypoglycemia.
SubChapter: Thermoregulation

Q316. Answer: A

Explanation: Feeding is appropriate for asymptomatic hypoglycemia to increase glucose availability and prevent CNS injury. IV therapy is reserved for symptomatic or persistent low values. Delaying recheck or failing to act can allow neuroglycopenia to develop.
SubChapter: Metabolic Assessment

Q317. Answer: B

Explanation: Temperature instability and feeding difficulty often appear first in sepsis due to metabolic and perfusion changes. Pink color and cry show well-being. Acrocyanosis and transient tachypnea are normal transitional findings.
SubChapter: Infection Assessment

Q318. Answer: B

Explanation: Absent Moro reflex may signify CNS injury or brachial plexus damage and requires immediate assessment. Tremors after crying and rooting/sucking are expected responses, while symmetry indicates normal motor function.
SubChapter: Neurologic Assessment

Q319. Answer: A

Explanation: Assessing intake helps determine whether oliguria is from inadequate feeding or renal issues. Intervention or notification follows only after data collection; catheterization or IV fluids may be unnecessary initially.
SubChapter: Renal Assessment

Q320. Answer: C

Explanation: A murmur lasting beyond 48 hours may indicate a cardiac defect like PDA or VSD and needs evaluation. Weight loss < 10 %, cord drying, and peeling skin are normal postnatal changes.
SubChapter: Cardiovascular Follow-Up

Q321. Answer: B

Explanation: Early breastfeeding transfers colostral IgA and immune factors that protect mucosal surfaces. Delayed feeding or isolation limits immunity, while early bathing removes vernix that offers microbial barrier benefits.
SubChapter: Immunologic Protection

Q322. Answer: B

Explanation: Petechiae outside pressure areas suggest thrombocytopenia or birth trauma requiring evaluation. Mongolian spots, milia, and erythema toxicum are benign pigment or immune findings.
SubChapter: Dermatologic Assessment

Q323. Answer: A

Explanation: Normal heart rate is 110–160, respirations 30–60, and temperature 97.7–99.5 °F. Lower rates indicate bradycardia; higher rates and fever suggest distress or infection.
SubChapter: Vital Signs Assessment

Q324. Answer: A

Explanation: Oxygen saturation > 95 % on room air indicates successful pulmonary adaptation. Cyanosis, apnea, and grunting represent distress requiring evaluation for hypoxia or RDS.
SubChapter: Respiratory Transition

Q325. Answer: B

Explanation: Wide fontanelle and sutures are associated with endocrine disorders like hypothyroidism or ICP from hydrocephalus. Dehydration causes sunken fontanelle; premature closure reduces size rather than expanding it.
SubChapter: Cranial Assessment

Q326. Answer: B

Explanation: Single umbilical artery can signal renal or cardiac anomalies; ultrasound screens for associated defects. Routine cleaning or clamping does not address possible underlying issues.
SubChapter: Anatomic Assessment

Q327. Answer: A

Explanation: Stable temperature and pink skin show effective thermogenesis. Newborns do not shiver; they use brown fat metabolism. Cool skin and apnea signify cold stress needing rewarming.
SubChapter: Thermoregulatory Assessment

Q328. Answer: A

Explanation: CCHD screening requires pre- and post-ductal pulse oximetry; a difference > 3 % or SpO_2 < 95 % needs evaluation. Auscultation alone misses silent defects. Refill and pulses support but do not replace screening.
SubChapter: Cardiac Screening

Q329. Answer: B

Explanation: The second reactive period (6–8 h post-birth) features alertness and feeding readiness, reflecting neurologic stability. Sleep and lethargy are normal in quiet phase, not reactivity. Hypothermia signifies stress, not adaptation.
SubChapter: Behavioral Adaptation

Q330. Answer: A

Explanation: Monitoring for bleeding and first void ensures hemostasis and urethral patency. Pressure dressings or alcohol cause tissue damage; bathing increases infection risk immediately post-procedure.
SubChapter: Post-Procedure Assessment

Q331. Answer: A

Explanation: Transient strabismus results from immature ocular muscles and resolves by 4 months. Purulent discharge suggests infection; cloudy cornea or absent red reflex require ophthalmic evaluation for cataracts or retinoblastoma.
SubChapter: Sensory Assessment

Q332. Answer: A

Explanation: Blood breakdown from cephalohematoma releases bilirubin, raising risk of jaundice. Infection or fracture is rare without open lesion or trauma. ICP remains unchanged in localized hematomas.
SubChapter: Hematologic Assessment

Q333. Answer: D
Explanation: Peripheral cyanosis with pink core shortly after birth is normal as circulation stabilizes. Central cyanosis or low SpO_2 would require oxygen or evaluation, but acrocyanosis alone is benign and transient.
SubChapter: Circulatory Transition
Q334. Answer: B
Explanation: Limited hip abduction with an audible click suggests developmental dysplasia of the hip and warrants orthopedic evaluation. Equal leg lengths and symmetric folds indicate normal alignment. Flexed posture and strong grasp are healthy neonatal tone findings.
SubChapter: Musculoskeletal Assessment
Q335. Answer: A
Explanation: A calm, pink newborn demonstrates stable temperature regulation and metabolic homeostasis. Jitteriness and cyanosis reflect cold stress or hypoglycemia, while weak cry and cool limbs indicate inadequate thermal balance requiring intervention.
SubChapter: Thermoregulation
Q336. Answer: A
Explanation: Distention with firmness may signal obstruction or delayed stool passage; auscultation and stool assessment guide diagnosis. Feeding or massage can worsen obstruction, and documentation alone ignores a potentially serious condition.
SubChapter: Gastrointestinal Assessment
Q337. Answer: B
Explanation: Hypoglycemia is the most frequent cause of neonatal jitteriness and poor feeding; prompt glucose evaluation prevents CNS injury. Bilirubin and calcium abnormalities present with different symptom patterns.
SubChapter: Metabolic Assessment
Q338. Answer: B
Explanation: A weak or absent suck reflex may indicate CNS depression, prematurity, or brain injury. Symmetry in Moro and flexed tone indicate normal neurologic integrity. Rooting is an expected feeding reflex.
SubChapter: Neurologic Function
Q339. Answer: A
Explanation: Peeling skin and decreased vernix reflect prolonged gestation and reduced amniotic fluid protection. Lanugo and soft cartilage are preterm features associated with immaturity rather than postmaturity.
SubChapter: Gestational Age Assessment
Q340. Answer: A
Explanation: Laryngomalacia causes intermittent inspiratory stridor due to soft supraglottic cartilage collapsing during inspiration, often resolving by 12–18 months. Other conditions present with severe respiratory distress and cyanosis, not mild intermittent stridor.
SubChapter: Airway Assessment
Q341. Answer: C
Explanation: Tachypnea with grunting indicates respiratory distress, possibly from infection or retained lung fluid, requiring immediate evaluation. Moist stump and slight irregular heart rate during sleep are normal, and 97.9 °F is within normal thermal limits.
SubChapter: Respiratory Distress
Q342. Answer: A

Explanation: Jaundice within 24 hours suggests pathologic hyperbilirubinemia from hemolysis or infection, requiring lab evaluation. Observation alone risks kernicterus. Feeding helps excretion but does not address cause; sunlight is unsafe for newborn therapy.
SubChapter: Hepatic Assessment
Q343. Answer: A
Explanation: Warm water and short exposure minimize evaporative and convective heat loss. Wet skin and immediate bathing increase hypothermia risk, while air drying without covering prolongs cooling.
SubChapter: Thermoregulation
Q344. Answer: A
Explanation: At least six wet diapers after day 4 confirm sufficient intake and hydration. Excess weight loss, absent stool, or dry mucosa imply feeding difficulties or dehydration needing lactation assessment.
SubChapter: Nutrition and Hydration
Q345. Answer: D
Explanation: Oxygen saturation < 90 % after 10 minutes indicates hypoxemia possibly due to congenital heart disease. Acrocyanosis and short murmurs are normal findings during transition.
SubChapter: Cardiovascular Screening
Q346. Answer: A
Explanation: Facial grimace with high-pitched cry indicates nociceptive response mediated by autonomic activation. Relaxed posture, stable heart rate, and sleep suggest comfort and pain relief.
SubChapter: Pain Assessment
Q347. Answer: A
Explanation: Diaphragmatic hernia causes abdominal organs to migrate into thoracic cavity, leading to scaphoid abdomen and respiratory distress. NEC and pyloric stenosis appear later; omphalocele is external at birth.
SubChapter: Gastrointestinal Assessment
Q348. Answer: A
Explanation: Axillary digital measurement is safe and reliable for neonates. Rectal and tympanic methods risk mucosal injury or inaccuracy; oral route is contraindicated in newborns.
SubChapter: Vital Signs Technique
Q349. Answer: D
Explanation: IUGR infants appear thin with loose skin and large fontanelle from reduced subcutaneous fat. Macrosomic infants exhibit excess fat. Vernix and lanugo reflect gestational age, not growth pattern.
SubChapter: Growth and Nutrition
Q350. Answer: A
Explanation: The Moro reflex is a startle response that protects from loss of support by triggering limb extension then flexion. Rooting aids feeding, Babinski indicates normal CNS, and stepping demonstrates motor tone only.
SubChapter: Neurologic Reflexes
Q351. Answer: A
Explanation: Functional foramen ovale closure occurs as left atrial pressure rises after birth, marking successful circulatory transition. Ductus patency, weak pulses, or cyanosis suggest cardiac pathology.
SubChapter: Cardiovascular Transition
Q352. Answer: A
Explanation: Preterm infants lack brown fat for thermogenesis and have high surface-to-mass ratio, making them prone to rapid heat loss. Term and LGA infants maintain better insulation and metabolic stability.
SubChapter: Thermoregulation
Q353. Answer: C

Explanation: Persistent hypoglycemia despite oral feeding requires IV dextrose to prevent neurologic injury. Warming and increased feeding alone cannot correct refractory low glucose. Early intervention ensures cerebral protection.
SubChapter: Metabolic Management
Q354. Answer: A
Explanation: An Apgar of 4 indicates inadequate breathing and bradycardia requiring ventilation to improve oxygenation. Compressions begin if heart rate stays < 60 bpm after ventilation. Temperature or glucose correction follows stabilization.
SubChapter: Immediate Post-Birth Care
Q355. Answer: A
Explanation: Vernix acts as a barrier against fluid loss and infection and is normal in creases. Generalized cyanosis, early jaundice, and petechiae suggest distress or pathology.
SubChapter: Integumentary Assessment
Q356. Answer: A
Explanation: High-pitched cry may indicate neurologic injury, intracranial pressure, or drug withdrawal. Hunger or overstimulation produce typical rhythmic cries, and congestion causes grunting or nasal sounds, not shrill tones.
SubChapter: Neurologic Assessment
Q357. Answer: D
Explanation: A flat, soft fontanelle at rest indicates normal hydration and pressure. Dehydration causes sunken fontanelle; bulging implies increased ICP. Anemia does not affect fontanelle tension.
SubChapter: Head Assessment
Q358. Answer: A
Explanation: Unequal Moro response indicates brachial plexus or clavicle injury. Jitteriness and acrocyanosis are transient adaptation signs, and irregular respirations are typical for quiet sleep.
SubChapter: Neuromuscular Assessment
Q359. Answer: A
Explanation: Elevated hematocrit (> 65%) indicates polycythemia, increasing blood viscosity and risk of hypoglycemia from increased metabolic demand. Hypocalcemia and infection are unrelated; anemia represents opposite imbalance.
SubChapter: Hematologic Assessment
Q360. Answer: A
Explanation: White, adherent plaques that resist wiping indicate oral candidiasis requiring antifungal treatment. Epstein pearls are benign cysts. Pink mucosa and strong suck reflect normal health.
SubChapter: Oral Assessment
Q361. Answer: D
Explanation: Urine output of 1–3 mL/kg/hr shows proper renal perfusion and function. Delayed void, crystals, or blood indicate dehydration or renal immaturity needing further evaluation.
SubChapter: Renal Assessment
Q362. Answer: A
Explanation: Excess red blood cell concentration causes ruddy skin tone, typical of polycythemia. Anemia results in pallor, while hypoxia causes cyanosis, and hypothermia gives a mottled appearance.
SubChapter: Circulatory Assessment
Q363. Answer: A
Explanation: Warming the heel promotes vasodilation, improving blood flow and minimizing pain. Deep or repeated punctures increase risk of tissue injury; the outer heel edge is the correct site.
SubChapter: Procedure Preparation
Q364. Answer: A

Explanation: Mild tremors with normal tone and feeding reflect immature neurologic control and are benign. Metabolic or infectious causes would present with poor tone, feeding, or abnormal vitals.
SubChapter: Neuromotor Assessment
Q365. Answer: D
Explanation: Mild tachypnea immediately post-birth likely reflects transient fluid clearance. Observation is appropriate if oxygenation remains stable. Persistent distress requires escalation, but early intervention without hypoxia may be unnecessary.
SubChapter: Respiratory Transition
Q366. Answer: A
Explanation: Universal screenings for hearing and CCHD detect silent anomalies before discharge. Vitamin K and vaccines are treatments, while education complements but doesn't replace essential screenings.
SubChapter: Discharge Readiness
Q367. Answer: A
Explanation: Grunting, retractions, and cyanosis indicate alveolar collapse and surfactant deficiency typical of RDS. Transient tachypnea and mild flaring are self-limited adjustment processes.
SubChapter: Respiratory Pathophysiology
Q368. Answer: A
Explanation: Immediate drying prevents fluid evaporation, the primary cause of early neonatal heat loss. Warm blankets reduce convective loss; avoiding metal reduces conductive loss; head covering helps later but not initially.
SubChapter: Thermoregulation
Q369. Answer: C
Explanation: Low glycogen or delayed feeding reduce energy substrate, leading to hypoglycemia. Bilirubin and calcium disturbances cause other symptoms; cold stress may worsen hypoglycemia but not cause it primarily.
SubChapter: Metabolic Assessment
Q370. Answer: A
Explanation: Uneven chest expansion often results from pneumothorax or musculoskeletal injury impairing ventilation. Transitional breathing affects both sides equally. Hernia causes severe distress and scaphoid abdomen.
SubChapter: Respiratory Assessment
Q371. Answer: A
Explanation: Capillary refill under 3 seconds confirms adequate perfusion and cardiac output. Heart rate and temperature alone don't measure tissue perfusion directly; blood pressure varies widely in neonates.
SubChapter: Circulatory Assessment
Q372. Answer: A
Explanation: Irregular breathing with no color change is typical during early neonatal adjustment. Grunting or pallor signals pathology, and hypothermia below 36 °C reflects thermal instability requiring correction.
SubChapter: Transitional Physiology
Q373. Answer: C
Explanation: Cold stress raises oxygen and glucose demands, predisposing to hypoglycemia and metabolic acidosis. Low respiratory effort, hyperglycemia, or seizures occur in other conditions, not mild cold exposure.
SubChapter: Thermoregulation
Q374. Answer: A

Explanation: Nasal flaring and retractions signal increased respiratory effort to maintain oxygenation. These findings require evaluation for respiratory distress syndrome or infection. Periodic breathing without retractions is normal, and overstimulation causes crying, not flaring.
SubChapter: Respiratory Assessment

Q375. Answer: A
Explanation: Infants of diabetic mothers experience excess insulin production from maternal hyperglycemia, predisposing them to rebound hypoglycemia after birth. SGA and preterm infants also risk low glucose but less predictably.
SubChapter: Metabolic Regulation

Q376. Answer: A
Explanation: Six or more wet diapers daily confirm good hydration and milk intake. A sunken fontanelle or dry mucosa indicates dehydration, and 12% weight loss exceeds the normal limit of 10%.
SubChapter: Fluid Balance

Q377. Answer: D
Explanation: Cold stress triggers non-shivering thermogenesis, consuming glucose and oxygen to produce heat, which can lead to hypoglycemia and acidosis. Metabolic rate increases, not decreases, during rewarming attempts.
SubChapter: Thermoregulation

Q378. Answer: C
Explanation: SpO_2 below 90% indicates inadequate oxygenation requiring evaluation for cardiac or pulmonary pathology. Mild murmurs and brief tachypnea may occur transiently in normal adaptation.
SubChapter: Oxygenation Assessment

Q379. Answer: A
Explanation: Polycythemia increases blood viscosity, producing ruddy skin, sluggish perfusion, and lethargy. Pallor suggests anemia; hypothermia and jitteriness relate to metabolic stress, not red cell excess.
SubChapter: Hematologic Assessment

Q380. Answer: A
Explanation: Skin-to-skin contact promotes conduction heat transfer and stabilizes vital signs, preventing cold stress. Delaying drying or early bathing increases evaporative loss. Swaddling helps later but not initially.
SubChapter: Thermoregulation

Q381. Answer: A
Explanation: Neonatal herpes spreads via direct contact; isolation prevents transmission. Jaundice and birth trauma lesions are noninfectious. Isolation is critical due to HSV's high morbidity in neonates.
SubChapter: Infection Control

Q382. Answer: C
Explanation: Jaundice developing after 24 hours is physiologic due to immature hepatic conjugation. Earlier onset or persistence > 7 days signals pathologic causes like hemolysis or obstruction.
SubChapter: Hepatic Function

Q383. Answer: A
Explanation: Absence of red reflex suggests cataract or retinoblastoma and requires urgent ophthalmologic referral. Other findings are benign birth or adaptation results.
SubChapter: Sensory Assessment

Q384. Answer: A
Explanation: Newborn respirations are irregular; a full 60-second count ensures accuracy. Counting for shorter intervals may miss pauses or tachypnea. Crying or post-feeding affects baseline rate.
SubChapter: Vital Signs Technique

Q385. Answer: A
Explanation: TTN results from delayed lung fluid absorption, common after cesarean birth. It presents with mild tachypnea and resolves within 48 hours. The other conditions cause severe distress and hypoxemia.
SubChapter: Respiratory Adaptation
Q386. Answer: C
Explanation: Startle followed by calm demonstrates intact sensory and neurologic response. Lack of reactivity or prolonged irritability may suggest CNS or metabolic disorders. Extended sleep interferes with feeding and indicates lethargy.
SubChapter: Behavioral Assessment
Q387. Answer: A
Explanation: $SpO_2 < 94\%$ after 10 minutes indicates hypoxemia needing oxygen support. Observation without correction risks desaturation; feeding increases oxygen demand and worsens hypoxia.
SubChapter: Oxygenation
Q388. Answer: A
Explanation: Apnea > 15 seconds with cyanosis suggests apnea of infancy or CNS dysfunction requiring immediate stimulation and evaluation. Other findings are benign and self-resolving.
SubChapter: Respiratory Pathophysiology
Q389. Answer: A
Explanation: Late preterm infants (34–36 weeks) exhibit smooth soles and soft cartilage, reflecting incomplete maturity. Firm cartilage and dry peeling skin indicate term or postterm status.
SubChapter: Gestational Maturity
Q390. Answer: C
Explanation: Eye contact during feeding demonstrates attachment and engagement, key for early bonding. Avoidance or delegation reflects adjustment difficulties or anxiety requiring support.
SubChapter: Family-Centered Care
Q391. Answer: A
Explanation: Temperature instability with respiratory distress are classic neonatal sepsis indicators needing cultures and antibiotics. Acrocyanosis and physiologic jaundice are normal, while 8% loss is acceptable adaptation.
SubChapter: Infection Recognition
Q392. Answer: A
Explanation: Hypocalcemia causes neuromuscular irritability, manifesting as jitteriness and shrill cry. Other symptoms occur in hypothermia, sepsis, or hypoglycemia but not isolated calcium deficiency.
SubChapter: Electrolyte Balance
Q393. Answer: A
Explanation: Hypothermia increases glucose utilization, leading to hypoglycemia; glucose should be checked promptly. Heart rate and color changes are secondary indicators, while urine output reflects later systemic effects.
SubChapter: Thermoregulation
Q394. Answer: C
Explanation: Central cyanosis indicates systemic hypoxemia and respiratory or cardiac compromise needing oxygen and evaluation. Acrocyanosis and mild irregular respirations are normal. Transient murmurs resolve as the ductus arteriosus closes.
SubChapter: Cardiopulmonary Assessment
Q395. Answer: A
Explanation: Cold stress manifests as mottled skin, lethargy, and weak cry due to peripheral vasoconstriction and energy depletion. Pink, warm skin and quiet alert state indicate thermal stability.

SubChapter: Thermoregulation

Q396. Answer: A

Explanation: Preterm infants lack sufficient surfactant, leading to alveolar collapse and RDS. Meconium aspiration causes obstruction, not RDS. Postterm and SGA infants face different complications.

SubChapter: Pulmonary Adaptation

Q397. Answer: A

Explanation: Strong pulses and heart rate within 110–160 bpm reflect effective cardiac transition. Cyanosis and delayed refill indicate poor perfusion or defect. Murmur with weak pulses suggests obstruction.

SubChapter: Cardiovascular Transition

Q398. Answer: C

Explanation: Conductive heat loss occurs from contact with cold objects; prewarmed blankets or surfaces prevent it. Drying prevents evaporative loss, radiant warmers counter convective loss, and hats reduce overall heat loss later.

SubChapter: Thermal Regulation

Q399. Answer: A

Explanation: Congenital hypothyroidism presents with macroglossia, wide fontanelle, and hypotonia from metabolic depression. Tremors and irritability suggest withdrawal; pale skin or tachypnea are unrelated systemic signs.

SubChapter: Endocrine Assessment

Q400. Answer: A

Explanation: Immediate stabilization follows the ABC sequence: airway, breathing, and temperature maintenance. Reflex assessment and prophylactic care follow after stabilization and Apgar scoring.

SubChapter: Immediate Newborn Care

Questions (401-500)

Q401. Which finding indicates pathologic jaundice?

A. Onset within 12 hours of birth
B. Peak bilirubin 8 mg/dL at 3 days
C. Resolution by 7 days
D. Limited to face and trunk

Q402. Which assessment finding is expected for a healthy term newborn?

A. HR 160, RR 70, temperature 97°F
B. HR 95, RR 25, temperature 96°F
C. HR 180, RR 80, temperature 100.8°F
D. RR 50, HR 130, temperature 98.6°F

Q403. Which observation during feeding indicates readiness to feed?

A. Coordinated sucking, swallowing, and breathing
B. Spitting and gagging
C. Decreased tone and weak suck
D. Cyanosis during feeding

Q404. A newborn presents with abdominal distention and no stool passage in 48 hours. Which condition should be suspected?

A. Hirschsprung disease
B. Necrotizing enterocolitis
C. Gastroesophageal reflux
D. Meconium plug syndrome

Q405. What is the correct interpretation of a newborn's hematocrit of 45%?
A. Normal value for term infant
B. Polycythemia
C. Anemia
D. Blood loss
Q406. Which assessment technique best evaluates newborn hip stability?
A. Observing leg movement only
B. Checking reflex symmetry
C. Ortolani and Barlow maneuvers
D. Measuring thigh circumference
Q407. Which finding suggests neonatal abstinence syndrome?
A. Tremors, shrill cry, poor feeding
B. Bradycardia, lethargy, hypotonia
C. Hypothermia and cyanosis
D. Quiet behavior and steady tone
Q408. Which condition is associated with a single umbilical artery?
A. Renal or cardiac malformation
B. Respiratory distress
C. Hyperbilirubinemia
D. Hypoglycemia
Q409. What finding differentiates cephalohematoma from caput succedaneum?
A. Caput indicates skull fracture
B. Cephalohematoma appears at birth and resolves in hours
C. Caput is confined to parietal bone
D. Cephalohematoma does not cross suture lines
Q410. Which newborn finding is considered abnormal?
A. SpO_2 87% after 10 minutes on room air
B. Acrocyanosis with pink trunk
C. Irregular respirations 35–55/min
D. HR 150 with crying
Q411. A woman develops sudden shortness of breath and chest pain 3 days after cesarean birth. Oxygen saturation is 86%. Which postpartum complication is most likely?
A. Pulmonary embolism
B. Pneumonia
C. Amniotic fluid embolism
D. Atelectasis
Q412. Two hours after vaginal delivery, a patient has heavy vaginal bleeding, a boggy uterus, and tachycardia. What is the priority nursing action?
A. Assess for lacerations
B. Massage the uterine fundus
C. Administer oxygen
D. Call for surgical evaluation
Q413. A woman presents 7 days postpartum with foul-smelling lochia, abdominal tenderness, and fever of 101.8°F (38.8°C). What condition is most likely?
A. Endometritis
B. Wound infection
C. Mastitis
D. Urinary tract infection

Q414. A postpartum woman with diabetes complains of excessive thirst, fatigue, and blurred vision. Blood glucose is 325 mg/dL. What is the most likely cause?
A. Hypoglycemia
B. Postpartum thyroiditis
C. Poor glycemic control
D. Adrenal insufficiency
Q415. Which finding best differentiates postpartum psychosis from postpartum depression?
A. Fatigue and insomnia
B. Persistent sadness
C. Delusional thinking
D. Loss of interest in activities
Q416. A woman develops fever, chills, and painful breast redness 10 days postpartum while breastfeeding. What is the appropriate nursing intervention?
A. Stop breastfeeding
B. Apply cold compresses
C. Continue breastfeeding and start antibiotics
D. Perform breast massage only
Q417. A postpartum patient has leg pain, warmth, and redness along the calf vein. What is the best immediate management?
A. Apply heat and encourage ambulation
B. Elevate the leg and notify the provider
C. Massage the area
D. Apply ice
Q418. A woman develops tremor, weight loss, anxiety, and tachycardia 4 weeks after delivery. Which disorder should be suspected?
A. Hypothyroidism
B. Postpartum thyroiditis (hyperthyroid phase)
C. Preeclampsia
D. Addison's disease
Q419. Six hours after cesarean birth, the patient reports dizziness and pallor. Vital signs show BP 82/50 mm Hg and HR 122 bpm. What is the priority action?
A. Assess incision
B. Administer IV fluids
C. Elevate the legs
D. Assess uterine tone
Q420. A woman complains of severe headache and visual disturbances 4 days postpartum. BP is 162/104 mm Hg. What diagnosis is most consistent?
A. Preeclampsia
B. Migraine
C. Hypoglycemia
D. Postpartum thyroiditis
Q421. A woman reports shortness of breath, cough with frothy sputum, and orthopnea two weeks postpartum. Auscultation reveals crackles. What is the likely diagnosis?
A. Postpartum cardiomyopathy
B. Pulmonary embolism
C. Pneumonia
D. Amniotic fluid embolism

Q422. After a difficult vaginal birth, a patient has perineal pain, swelling, and a firm 4-cm bluish mass near the vaginal opening. What complication is suspected?
A. Hematoma
B. Laceration infection
C. Varicosity
D. Cystocele
Q423. A postpartum client presents with fever, tachycardia, and foul discharge after cesarean section. The incision appears intact. Which organism commonly causes this?
A. Staphylococcus aureus
B. Escherichia coli
C. Streptococcus pyogenes
D. Klebsiella pneumoniae
Q424. Which lab pattern supports a diagnosis of disseminated intravascular coagulation (DIC) following postpartum hemorrhage?
A. Elevated fibrinogen and platelets
B. Prolonged PT/aPTT, low fibrinogen, low platelets
C. Normal coagulation profile
D. Isolated elevated hematocrit
Q425. A woman 3 days postpartum develops right upper quadrant pain, fever, and mild jaundice after prolonged labor. Which diagnosis is most likely?
A. Gallbladder disease
B. Hepatic vein thrombosis
C. Hepatitis B infection
D. Preeclampsia
Q426. Five days after birth, a patient develops high fever and localized erythema around her cesarean incision with purulent drainage. Which nursing action is priority?
A. Apply topical ointment
B. Notify provider for wound culture
C. Cover with ice packs
D. Leave wound open to air
Q427. A mother reports sadness, poor concentration, and inability to bond with her infant for over 3 weeks. She denies hallucinations. What is the most likely diagnosis?
A. Postpartum blues
B. Postpartum depression
C. Postpartum psychosis
D. Adjustment disorder
Q428. A postpartum patient reports numbness and tingling in the hands. Trousseau's sign is positive. Which complication is indicated?
A. Hypocalcemia after PPH
B. Hypoglycemia
C. Carpal tunnel syndrome
D. Preeclampsia
Q429. Two weeks postpartum, a woman develops severe anxiety about her infant's safety, repeatedly checking on the baby, yet recognizes her thoughts as excessive. What condition is likely?
A. Postpartum depression
B. Postpartum obsessive–compulsive disorder
C. Psychosis
D. Generalized anxiety disorder

Q430. A postpartum woman complains of fever, dysuria, and flank pain. Urinalysis shows leukocytes and nitrites. What is the correct diagnosis?
A. Cystitis
B. Pyelonephritis
C. Ureteral trauma
D. Pelvic abscess
Q431. A patient experiences heavy bleeding 10 days after delivery. The uterus feels firm and midline. Which condition should be suspected?
A. Uterine atony
B. Retained placental fragments
C. Coagulation disorder
D. Cervical laceration
Q432. Which nursing finding is most concerning for a woman at risk for postpartum hemorrhage?
A. Saturating one pad every two hours
B. Fundus firm, one centimeter below umbilicus
C. Heart rate 120 bpm and pallor
D. Moderate lochia rubra on day 2
Q433. A 3-day postpartum client reports chills, malaise, and localized breast tenderness without systemic toxicity. What should the nurse recommend?
A. Stop breastfeeding temporarily
B. Apply cold compresses only
C. Continue breastfeeding and apply warm compresses
D. Begin prophylactic antibiotics
Q434. A patient reports extreme sadness, loss of appetite, and hopelessness beginning one month after birth. She denies suicidal thoughts. What is the best initial intervention?
A. Provide reassurance it is normal
B. Encourage counseling and mental health referral
C. Increase iron intake
D. Recommend more rest and fluids
Q435. Following a cesarean delivery, a patient develops persistent tachycardia and hypoxia with clear lungs on auscultation. What is the nurse's immediate concern?
A. Fluid overload
B. Pulmonary embolism
C. Atelectasis
D. Heart failure
Q436. Which postpartum finding requires urgent follow-up?
A. Lochia serosa on day five
B. Temperature 100.2°F once on day two
C. Foul-smelling lochia and uterine tenderness
D. Firm fundus at umbilicus
Q437. A postpartum woman presents with confusion, agitation, and auditory hallucinations three days after delivery. What is the priority nursing action?
A. Provide sleep and hydration
B. Contact the healthcare provider immediately
C. Suggest outpatient counseling
D. Reassure the family
Q438. A woman experiences severe perineal pain unrelieved by analgesics, with swelling and bluish discoloration. Vital signs show mild tachycardia. Which is the likely diagnosis?

A. Perineal infection
B. Hematoma
C. Laceration
D. Edema

Q439. A patient one week postpartum reports urinary frequency, burning, and suprapubic pain. Which finding confirms the diagnosis?

A. Cloudy urine with bacteria and leukocytes
B. High blood pressure and proteinuria
C. Vaginal discharge
D. Normal urinalysis

Q440. A postpartum patient with heavy bleeding receives oxytocin and fundal massage without improvement. Which medication should be given next?

A. Terbutaline
B. Methylergonovine
C. Magnesium sulfate
D. Hydralazine

Q441. A patient with postpartum hemorrhage receives several units of blood. Later, she develops oozing from IV sites and low fibrinogen levels. Which condition is this?

A. Thrombocytopenia
B. DIC secondary to transfusion reaction
C. Sepsis
D. Hemophilia

Q442. Which finding indicates successful management of postpartum hemorrhage after uterotonics?

A. Saturating pads every 30 minutes
B. Firm, midline fundus with scant lochia
C. Persistent hypotension
D. Clots larger than 3 cm

Q443. Which postpartum client is most at risk for venous thromboembolism?

A. Vaginal delivery without complications
B. Cesarean birth with prolonged bed rest
C. Early ambulation after birth
D. Multiparity without medical history

Q444. A postpartum woman presents with fever and right breast pain localized to one area, but she is able to continue breastfeeding. What is the diagnosis?

A. Mastitis
B. Plugged duct
C. Abscess
D. Fibrocystic change

Q445. A woman develops confusion, severe headache, and blood pressure of 170/110 mm Hg on the second postpartum day. Which treatment is indicated?

A. Diuretic therapy only
B. Magnesium sulfate and antihypertensives
C. Fluid restriction only
D. Oxytocin infusion

Q446. A patient presents two weeks postpartum with depression, fatigue, and inability to sleep even when the baby rests. Which statement reflects appropriate nursing care?

A. Encourage counseling and evaluate for antidepressant therapy
B. Advise to wait for symptoms to pass naturally

C. Suggest more iron and fluids
D. Recommend avoiding visitors until mood improves

Q447. Which patient is most at risk for postpartum infection?
A. Cesarean delivery after prolonged rupture of membranes
B. Rapid vaginal birth
C. Planned cesarean without labor
D. First-degree perineal tear

Q448. A postpartum woman exhibits fatigue, dry skin, and weight gain six months after delivery. Which condition is likely?
A. Postpartum thyroiditis (hypothyroid phase)
B. Cushing syndrome
C. Addison's disease
D. Type 1 diabetes mellitus

Q449. A mother with mastitis fails to improve after 48 hours of antibiotics and develops fluctuating swelling with pus drainage. What is the next step?
A. Continue oral antibiotics only
B. Apply warm compresses
C. Perform incision and drainage
D. Discontinue breastfeeding permanently

Q450. A patient with severe postpartum hemorrhage receives methylergonovine but develops a headache and BP 170/108 mm Hg. What should the nurse do next?
A. Continue the medication
B. Discontinue drug and notify provider immediately
C. Give another dose for control
D. Document as expected effect

Q451. A woman experiences sharp chest pain and dyspnea two weeks postpartum. Oxygen saturation is 84%, and she is tachycardic. What is the immediate nursing action?
A. Place the patient flat in bed
B. Elevate the head and apply oxygen
C. Administer methylergonovine
D. Encourage ambulation

Q452. A postpartum client has a temperature of 101.5°F, uterine tenderness, and foul-smelling lochia on day four after cesarean birth. Which nursing priority applies?
A. Administer broad-spectrum antibiotics as prescribed
B. Encourage increased fluid intake only
C. Reassure that fever is normal
D. Apply warm compresses to abdomen

Q453. Which patient should avoid methylergonovine for postpartum hemorrhage management?
A. Diabetic
B. Hypertensive
C. Asthmatic
D. Primiparous

Q454. A woman complains of anxiety, restlessness, and feeling "disconnected" from reality five days after birth. She has auditory hallucinations. What should the nurse do first?
A. Notify the healthcare provider immediately
B. Encourage sleep and relaxation
C. Advise increased fluids
D. Suggest family support groups

Q455. A patient who experienced severe postpartum hemorrhage now shows extreme fatigue, pallor, and low hemoglobin. What therapy is expected?
A. IV oxytocin
B. Oral iron supplementation
C. Magnesium sulfate
D. Methylergonovine
Q456. Which finding indicates postpartum wound dehiscence after cesarean section?
A. Pink incision with mild tenderness
B. Fever 99°F with intact sutures
C. Separation of incision with serous drainage
D. Small hematoma near incision edge
Q457. A postpartum client develops seizures one week after birth. She previously had mild hypertension. Which condition is most likely?
A. Eclampsia
B. Hypoglycemia
C. Anxiety disorder
D. Postpartum psychosis
Q458. A woman reports severe right calf pain and swelling two weeks after cesarean delivery. Which diagnostic test should be anticipated?
A. Chest X-ray
B. Doppler ultrasound of leg veins
C. ECG
D. CBC with differential
Q459. Which symptom most strongly suggests postpartum depression rather than normal adjustment?
A. Tearfulness for two days
B. Fatigue relieved by rest
C. Persistent guilt and hopelessness for three weeks
D. Mood swings that resolve with support
Q460. A woman presents three weeks postpartum with pelvic pain, fever, and malodorous vaginal discharge. Ultrasound reveals retained tissue. What is the appropriate management?
A. Expectant observation
B. Dilation and curettage with antibiotics
C. Oxytocin infusion only
D. Iron therapy alone
Q461. A postpartum patient develops shortness of breath and hemoptysis on day 10 after cesarean birth. Her leg is swollen and tender. What complication should be suspected?
A. Pneumonia
B. Pulmonary embolism
C. Heart failure
D. Atelectasis
Q462. A nurse notes bright red bleeding and a firm uterus two hours after delivery. What is the most likely cause?
A. Retained placental fragments
B. Vaginal laceration
C. Uterine atony
D. DIC
Q463. A woman presents with breast pain, fever, and induration despite continued breastfeeding. What is the next best nursing action?

A. Stop breastfeeding immediately
B. Apply ice packs only
C. Notify provider; start antibiotics
D. Pump and discard milk

Q464. Which sign differentiates postpartum blues from postpartum depression?
A. Sadness that resolves in less than two weeks
B. Insomnia and crying episodes
C. Appetite changes and fatigue
D. Difficulty bonding with infant lasting over one month

Q465. A woman experiences recurrent fainting and pallor after severe postpartum hemorrhage. Laboratory values show low hemoglobin and hematocrit. Which complication is most likely?
A. Pulmonary embolism
B. Iron deficiency anemia
C. Endometritis
D. Preeclampsia

Q466. A postpartum woman develops high fever, flank pain, and costovertebral tenderness. Urinalysis reveals bacteria and white blood cells. What is the likely diagnosis?
A. Cystitis
B. Pyelonephritis
C. Endometritis
D. Pelvic abscess

Q467. A woman reports intense fear of harming her baby but recognizes the thoughts as irrational. She avoids caring for the infant. Which diagnosis fits best?
A. Postpartum psychosis
B. Postpartum obsessive–compulsive disorder
C. Postpartum depression
D. Panic disorder

Q468. A postpartum woman reports pain and swelling at her cesarean incision with foul drainage and fever. What is the most appropriate initial nursing action?
A. Cover with a dry dressing
B. Reassure and observe
C. Apply heat to the area
D. Obtain wound culture and notify provider

Q469. Which postpartum finding indicates possible thromboembolic disease?
A. Slight ankle edema bilaterally
B. Positive Homan's sign with calf tenderness
C. Cool extremities and pale color
D. Diminished pedal pulses bilaterally

Q470. A postpartum patient experiences persistent perineal pain with a purulent discharge from the episiotomy site. What should the nurse expect the provider to order?
A. Sitz baths only
B. Oral antibiotics and wound care
C. Topical cream
D. Observation without treatment

Q471. A patient develops chills, fever, and uterine tenderness on postpartum day 3 after prolonged rupture of membranes. Which organism is most commonly responsible?
A. Escherichia coli
B. Staphylococcus aureus

C. Chlamydia trachomatis
D. Pseudomonas aeruginosa

Q472. After cesarean birth, a patient experiences redness, warmth, and tenderness along her calf. What is the priority nursing action?

A. Encourage ambulation
B. Apply compression bandages
C. Place the leg on bed rest and notify the provider
D. Massage the area to improve circulation

Q473. A postpartum woman complains of extreme fatigue, dizziness, and pale skin. Her hemoglobin is 8 g/dL. What nursing intervention is appropriate?

A. Encourage increased fluid intake
B. Recommend dietary iron and supplements
C. Restrict physical activity completely
D. Administer oxytocin infusion

Q474. A postpartum woman has headache, blurred vision, and blood pressure of 160/100 mm Hg five days after delivery. Which diagnosis is most likely?

A. Postpartum thyroiditis
B. Postpartum preeclampsia
C. Depression
D. Hypoglycemia

Q475. A patient two weeks postpartum reports severe sadness, fatigue, and loss of interest in caring for her baby. Which intervention is appropriate?

A. Monitor symptoms for another week
B. Encourage professional mental health evaluation
C. Advise increased sleep and fluids
D. Reassure that emotional changes are normal

Q476. Which sign most strongly suggests retained placental fragments after delivery?

A. Foul-smelling lochia
B. Firm fundus with unexpected heavy bleeding
C. Low-grade fever
D. Perineal hematoma

Q477. A postpartum woman presents with a painful, fluctuant breast mass and fever after prior mastitis. What management is expected?

A. Needle aspiration or incision and drainage
B. Continue oral antibiotics only
C. Apply ice packs continuously
D. Cease all breastfeeding immediately

Q478. A postpartum client with a history of gestational diabetes presents with excessive thirst and fatigue. Blood glucose is 310 mg/dL. Which complication is suspected?

A. Postpartum hypoglycemia
B. Type 2 diabetes mellitus
C. Postpartum thyroiditis
D. Iron deficiency anemia

Q479. A woman reports persistent crying, irritability, and hopelessness two weeks after childbirth. Which statement differentiates her condition from baby blues?

A. Symptoms are self-limiting
B. Onset within the first 48 hours
C. Lasting more than two weeks and interfering with function

D. Alternating joy and sadness

Q480. A postpartum patient has generalized edema, proteinuria, and elevated blood pressure two weeks after delivery. What potential complication must be prevented?

A. Sepsis
B. Eclampsia
C. Pulmonary embolism
D. DIC

Q481. A postpartum woman develops severe shortness of breath, crackles, and pink frothy sputum one week after birth. She has no prior cardiac history. What should be suspected?

A. Pulmonary embolism
B. Postpartum cardiomyopathy
C. Pneumonia
D. Amniotic fluid embolism

Q482. A woman reports foul-smelling lochia, fever, and uterine tenderness on day six postpartum. Which assessment finding confirms infection?

A. Decreasing lochia flow
B. Soft, non-tender fundus
C. Elevated white blood cell count with left shift
D. Normal temperature after fluids

Q483. Which symptom is most consistent with postpartum depression?

A. Sudden onset of hallucinations
B. Excessive happiness alternating with sadness
C. Persistent sadness and inability to care for self or infant
D. Fatigue improving with rest

Q484. A woman's uterus remains firm but lochia becomes bright red and excessive on postpartum day seven. Which cause is likely?

A. Uterine atony
B. Retained placental fragments
C. Endometritis
D. Vaginal hematoma

Q485. A postpartum woman develops right calf swelling, redness, and pain. What intervention is appropriate while awaiting confirmation?

A. Elevate the leg and maintain bed rest
B. Apply warm compresses and massage
C. Encourage ambulation
D. Use elastic stockings immediately

Q486. A patient reports feeling overwhelmed, tearful, and anxious for one week after birth but continues to care for her baby. What condition is most likely?

A. Postpartum blues
B. Postpartum depression
C. Psychosis
D. Anxiety disorder

Q487. A postpartum patient who received large volumes of IV fluids now has dyspnea, crackles, and jugular distension. What is the suspected cause?

A. Pulmonary embolism
B. Fluid overload
C. Pneumonia
D. Endometritis

Q488. Which symptom suggests thyroid dysfunction after childbirth?
A. Tremors, anxiety, and weight loss
B. Dizziness and low blood pressure
C. Night sweats and breast tenderness
D. Constipation and uterine cramping
Q489. A woman with mastitis is prescribed antibiotics. What instruction should the nurse provide?
A. Stop breastfeeding until infection resolves
B. Continue breastfeeding or pumping frequently
C. Use cold compresses only
D. Avoid emptying the affected breast
Q490. A postpartum patient reports sharp perineal pain and pressure. Exam reveals a firm, swollen, purple mass near the vaginal opening. What should the nurse suspect?
A. Perineal infection
B. Vaginal hematoma
C. Laceration
D. Normal healing
Q491. A woman reports heavy bleeding and dizziness one week after delivery. The uterus is firm and non-tender. What is the likely cause?
A. Uterine atony
B. Retained placental tissue
C. Infection
D. Cervical laceration
Q492. Which postpartum finding most strongly suggests pulmonary embolism?
A. Low-grade fever and cough
B. Sudden dyspnea and chest pain
C. Crackles with pink frothy sputum
D. Bradycardia and hypotension
Q493. A patient complains of feeling sad, hopeless, and unable to sleep even when her baby rests. Symptoms began three weeks ago. Which action is best?
A. Encourage counseling and mental health evaluation
B. Recommend more rest and fluids
C. Reassure this is normal adjustment
D. Increase activity level
Q494. A postpartum client presents with high fever, chills, and purulent drainage from her cesarean incision. What is the initial nursing action?
A. Apply ice to reduce swelling
B. Obtain wound culture and notify provider
C. Continue routine wound care
D. Encourage ambulation
Q495. A woman with severe preeclampsia delivered two days ago. She now complains of headache and visual changes. What is the most important medication to continue?
A. Oxytocin
B. Magnesium sulfate
C. Terbutaline
D. Methylergonovine
Q496. A postpartum woman develops localized warmth and redness at her breast with flu-like symptoms. What should the nurse teach her?
A. Stop breastfeeding until antibiotics are finished

B. Continue feeding and apply warm compresses
C. Use tight bras to reduce milk flow
D. Express milk and discard it

Q497. A woman experiences fatigue, cold intolerance, and weight gain two months postpartum. Which disorder is likely?

A. Postpartum thyroiditis (hypothyroid phase)
B. Diabetes mellitus
C. Preeclampsia
D. Postpartum depression

Q498. A postpartum client with retained placenta develops oozing at IV sites and bleeding gums. What complication should the nurse suspect?

A. Endometritis
B. Disseminated intravascular coagulation
C. Anemia
D. Pulmonary embolism

Q499. A postpartum woman reports extreme mood swings, confusion, and auditory hallucinations four days after delivery. What should the nurse do first?

A. Provide reassurance and monitor
B. Notify provider immediately and ensure safety
C. Encourage rest and nutrition
D. Ask family to provide support

Q500. A woman complains of burning on urination and suprapubic pain five days postpartum. Urinalysis shows leukocytes and bacteria. Which is the appropriate management?

A. Encourage hydration and start antibiotics
B. Restrict fluids
C. Observe without treatment
D. Apply warm compresses to the abdomen

Answer key and Explanation (401-500)

Q401. Answer: A
Explanation: Jaundice appearing within 24 hours signifies hemolytic disease or infection. Physiologic jaundice peaks later and resolves by one week. Localized discoloration without early onset is benign.
SubChapter: Hepatic Function

Q402. Answer: D
Explanation: Normal newborn vitals include HR 110–160, RR 30–60, and temperature 97.7–99.5°F. Bradycardia, tachypnea, or hypothermia indicate abnormal adaptation.
SubChapter: Vital Signs Assessment

Q403. Answer: A
Explanation: Coordinated suck-swallow-breathe sequence demonstrates neurologic maturity and feeding readiness. Gagging, weak tone, or cyanosis indicate poor coordination and risk for aspiration.
SubChapter: Feeding Readiness

Q404. Answer: A
Explanation: Failure to pass meconium within 48 hours with distention suggests Hirschsprung disease due to absence of ganglion cells. NEC and reflux appear later; meconium plug usually resolves spontaneously.
SubChapter: Gastrointestinal Assessment

Q405. Answer: A
Explanation: Normal hematocrit for term infants ranges from 45–65%. Values below 40% indicate anemia, and above 65% reflect polycythemia. This level demonstrates healthy erythropoiesis.
SubChapter: Hematologic Assessment

Q406. Answer: C
Explanation: Ortolani and Barlow maneuvers detect hip dislocation by identifying joint clicks or instability. Reflex checks or leg movement alone cannot confirm hip dysplasia.
SubChapter: Musculoskeletal Assessment

Q407. Answer: A
Explanation: NAS presents with CNS irritability, including tremors, high-pitched cry, and feeding difficulties due to withdrawal. Bradycardia and lethargy indicate other metabolic issues.
SubChapter: Neurologic Assessment

Q408. Answer: A
Explanation: Single umbilical artery correlates with renal and cardiovascular anomalies; evaluation is warranted. Other conditions are unrelated to cord vessel abnormalities.
SubChapter: Anatomic Assessment

Q409. Answer: D
Explanation: Cephalohematoma, a subperiosteal bleed, is limited by sutures and appears hours post-delivery. Caput crosses sutures and resolves quickly; neither indicates fracture.
SubChapter: Birth Trauma Assessment

Q410. Answer: A
Explanation: Oxygen saturation below 90% after 10 minutes signals hypoxia and requires evaluation. Acrocyanosis and variable respirations are normal transitions; HR of 150 during crying is expected.
SubChapter: Oxygenation Assessment

Q411. Answer: A
Explanation: Pulmonary embolism is a leading postpartum cause of acute respiratory distress within the first week due to hypercoagulability and venous stasis. Option B is gradual in onset with fever; C occurs intrapartum or immediately postpartum; D causes mild, transient hypoxia without chest pain.
SubChapter: Cardiopulmonary & Thromboembolic Complications

Q412. Answer: B

Explanation: Uterine atony is the most common cause of postpartum hemorrhage. Immediate firm fundal massage stimulates uterine contraction and constricts open vessels. Option A follows if tone is normal; C supports oxygenation but does not treat the cause; D is indicated if conservative measures fail.

SubChapter: Hematologic & Hemorrhagic Disorders

Q413. Answer: A

Explanation: Postpartum endometritis typically develops within the first week after delivery due to ascending bacterial infection of the uterine lining. Foul odor, uterine tenderness, and fever are classic. Option B presents with localized wound redness; C involves breast pain and erythema; D features urinary urgency or flank pain rather than uterine tenderness.

SubChapter: Infectious Conditions

Q414. Answer: C

Explanation: Poor glycemic control in the postpartum period occurs due to altered insulin sensitivity, infection, or inadequate medication. Option A presents with diaphoresis and tremors; B causes fatigue and weight changes without hyperglycemia; D is rare and marked by hypotension and electrolyte imbalance.

SubChapter: Metabolic & Endocrine Disorders

Q415. Answer: C

Explanation: Delusions or hallucinations define postpartum psychosis, typically emerging within two weeks after birth, requiring emergency psychiatric intervention. Option A and B indicate depression or normal fatigue; D reflects anhedonia typical of depression, not psychosis. Prompt evaluation prevents harm to mother and infant.

SubChapter: Psychological & Neurologic Conditions

Q416. Answer: C

Explanation: Mastitis results from milk stasis and bacterial infection, often due to Staphylococcus aureus. Continuing breastfeeding aids drainage, while antibiotics resolve infection. Option A worsens engorgement; B provides temporary relief but does not address infection; D alone is inadequate.

SubChapter: Infectious Conditions

Q417. Answer: B

Explanation: These findings suggest superficial thrombophlebitis. Leg elevation promotes venous return and reduces swelling while awaiting evaluation. Option A risks embolization; C is contraindicated; D may reduce pain but not treat the thrombus.

SubChapter: Cardiopulmonary & Thromboembolic Complications

Q418. Answer: B

Explanation: Postpartum thyroiditis begins with a transient hyperthyroid phase followed by hypothyroidism. Option A presents later with fatigue and cold intolerance; C resolves after birth and does not cause weight loss; D features hypotension and hyperpigmentation, not tachycardia.

SubChapter: Metabolic & Endocrine Disorders

Q419. Answer: D

Explanation: Hypotension and tachycardia shortly after delivery strongly suggest hemorrhage from uterine atony. Assessing uterine tone identifies the cause and guides management before fluid resuscitation. Option B supports circulation but does not control bleeding; C provides temporary perfusion; A may detect external bleeding but not internal uterine loss.

SubChapter: Hematologic & Hemorrhagic Disorders

Q420. Answer: A

Explanation: Postpartum preeclampsia presents within six weeks of birth, featuring hypertension, headache, and visual symptoms. It may progress to eclampsia if untreated. Option B lacks hypertension;

C causes diaphoresis and confusion; D presents with fatigue, not elevated BP. Prompt magnesium sulfate and antihypertensive therapy prevent seizures.
SubChapter: Cardiopulmonary & Thromboembolic Complications

Q421. Answer: A

Explanation: Peripartum or postpartum cardiomyopathy manifests within months of delivery due to ventricular dysfunction. Dyspnea, orthopnea, and pulmonary congestion are typical. Option B presents acutely with pleuritic pain; C features fever and localized crackles; D occurs during or immediately after delivery with cardiovascular collapse rather than progressive dyspnea.
SubChapter: Cardiopulmonary & Thromboembolic Complications

Q422. Answer: A

Explanation: A vulvar hematoma results from vessel rupture and blood accumulation causing pain and tense swelling. Option B shows erythema and fever; C is soft and chronic; D is a pelvic organ prolapse, not an acute postpartum finding.
SubChapter: Hematologic & Hemorrhagic Disorders

Q423. Answer: B

Explanation: E. coli frequently causes endometritis after cesarean due to ascending contamination from the lower genital tract. Option A is typical of wound or breast infections; C produces severe systemic toxic shock; D is less common. Broad-spectrum antibiotics covering aerobic and anaerobic flora are indicated.
SubChapter: Infectious Conditions

Q424. Answer: B

Explanation: DIC involves consumption of clotting factors, yielding prolonged PT/aPTT, decreased fibrinogen, and thrombocytopenia. Option A is opposite of expected; C rules out DIC; D may indicate hemoconcentration but not coagulopathy. Management targets the underlying cause and supportive transfusion therapy.
SubChapter: Hematologic & Hemorrhagic Disorders

Q425. Answer: A

Explanation: Gallbladder stasis and stones are common postpartum due to hormonal effects on bile flow, causing RUQ pain and low-grade fever. Option B is rare; C presents with malaise and marked transaminase elevation; D occurs with hypertension, not isolated RUQ tenderness.
SubChapter: Metabolic & Endocrine Disorders

Q426. Answer: B

Explanation: Wound infection following cesarean requires prompt culture and systemic antibiotics. Option A is inadequate for deep infection; C may reduce swelling but delays diagnosis; D increases contamination risk. Early intervention prevents wound dehiscence and systemic spread.
SubChapter: Infectious Conditions

Q427. Answer: B

Explanation: Symptoms persisting beyond two weeks suggest postpartum depression, a mood disorder requiring therapy. Option A resolves within two weeks; C includes delusions or hallucinations; D is mild and short-term. Screening and early treatment improve maternal–infant outcomes.
SubChapter: Psychological & Neurologic Conditions

Q428. Answer: A

Explanation: Hypocalcemia may follow massive blood transfusion or DIC treatment where citrate binds calcium, causing neuromuscular irritability. Option B causes confusion, not tetany; C develops gradually during pregnancy; D includes hypertension and edema, not tetany. Calcium replacement resolves symptoms.
SubChapter: Metabolic & Endocrine Disorders

Q429. Answer: B

Explanation: Postpartum OCD features intrusive thoughts and repetitive checking behaviors but intact insight. It differs from psychosis, where reality testing is lost. Depression lacks compulsions, and generalized anxiety involves broader, non-specific worry. Cognitive-behavioral therapy and SSRIs are effective treatments.
SubChapter: Psychological & Neurologic Conditions
Q430. Answer: B
Explanation: Pyelonephritis involves upper urinary tract infection with fever and flank pain caused by ascending bacteria, usually E. coli. Option A lacks systemic symptoms; C presents immediately after surgery with hematuria; D causes localized pelvic tenderness without urinary findings. Prompt IV antibiotics are essential.
SubChapter: Infectious Conditions
Q431. Answer: B
Explanation: Late postpartum hemorrhage with a firm uterus often indicates retained placental tissue that maintains vascular patency. Atony causes a soft uterus, coagulation disorders cause oozing without localized source, and cervical lacerations bleed immediately after birth, not days later.
SubChapter: Hematologic & Hemorrhagic Disorders
Q432. Answer: C
Explanation: Tachycardia and pallor signal compensatory response to significant blood loss, even before visible hemorrhage. Normal lochia and uterine position suggest stable postpartum recovery. Pad counts are helpful but less sensitive than vital sign changes for detecting concealed bleeding.
SubChapter: Hematologic & Hemorrhagic Disorders
Q433. Answer: C
Explanation: Early milk stasis causes localized inflammation; frequent breastfeeding and warm compresses enhance milk flow and prevent infection. Stopping feeds worsens stasis, antibiotics are premature without infection, and cold compresses do not resolve obstruction.
SubChapter: Infectious Conditions
Q434. Answer: B
Explanation: Postpartum depression requires early psychological evaluation and support to prevent worsening symptoms. It differs from normal adjustment or "baby blues." Nutritional and rest recommendations alone do not address the mood disorder. Prompt therapy improves maternal bonding and safety.
SubChapter: Psychological & Neurologic Conditions
Q435. Answer: B
Explanation: Tachycardia, dyspnea, and low oxygen saturation with normal breath sounds suggest pulmonary embolism, a life-threatening postpartum complication. Atelectasis presents with diminished sounds; heart failure shows crackles; fluid overload causes wheezing and edema. Urgent evaluation and anticoagulation are critical.
SubChapter: Cardiopulmonary & Thromboembolic Complications
Q436. Answer: C
Explanation: Foul odor and uterine tenderness signify endometritis, a serious uterine infection. Lochia serosa and firm fundus are expected, and a single low-grade fever is common from dehydration or milk letdown. Prompt antibiotic therapy prevents sepsis.
SubChapter: Infectious Conditions
Q437. Answer: B
Explanation: Postpartum psychosis is a psychiatric emergency that requires immediate provider notification and possible hospitalization for safety. Rest and reassurance are insufficient and delay treatment. Early intervention prevents maternal or infant harm.
SubChapter: Psychological & Neurologic Conditions

Q438. Answer: B
Explanation: A tense, discolored perineal swelling unrelieved by medication indicates hematoma formation from vessel rupture. Infection develops later with redness and fever; lacerations bleed externally; simple edema causes less pain and discoloration.
SubChapter: Hematologic & Hemorrhagic Disorders
Q439. Answer: A
Explanation: Cloudy urine containing bacteria and leukocytes confirms cystitis, a common postpartum urinary infection. Hypertension and proteinuria suggest preeclampsia; vaginal discharge indicates reproductive tract infection; normal urinalysis excludes infection. Oral antibiotics and hydration are indicated.
SubChapter: Infectious Conditions
Q440. Answer: B
Explanation: Methylergonovine is administered after oxytocin if uterine atony persists, promoting sustained contraction to control bleeding. It is contraindicated in hypertension. Terbutaline relaxes the uterus; magnesium sulfate prevents seizures; hydralazine treats hypertension, not hemorrhage.
SubChapter: Hematologic & Hemorrhagic Disorders
Q441. Answer: B
Explanation: Disseminated intravascular coagulation follows massive transfusion or obstetric trauma, causing widespread clotting and bleeding. Low fibrinogen, prolonged PT/aPTT, and bleeding at puncture sites confirm the diagnosis. Thrombocytopenia alone shows low platelets but normal coagulation; sepsis presents with fever; hemophilia is hereditary and rare postpartum.
SubChapter: Hematologic & Hemorrhagic Disorders
Q442. Answer: B
Explanation: A firm, midline fundus and light bleeding confirm effective uterine contraction and hemostasis. Excessive pad use or large clots indicate continued bleeding, and hypotension suggests unresolved volume loss requiring further intervention.
SubChapter: Hematologic & Hemorrhagic Disorders
Q443. Answer: B
Explanation: Cesarean section combined with immobility significantly increases risk of thromboembolism from venous stasis and endothelial injury. Vaginal birth and ambulation protect against clot formation. Multiparity alone is not a strong independent risk factor.
SubChapter: Cardiopulmonary & Thromboembolic Complications
Q444. Answer: A
Explanation: Mastitis is characterized by localized breast pain, warmth, and fever, typically due to S. aureus. Continued breastfeeding helps drainage. A plugged duct lacks systemic symptoms; abscess involves fluctuance and purulent drainage; fibrocystic changes occur unrelated to lactation.
SubChapter: Infectious Conditions
Q445. Answer: B
Explanation: Postpartum preeclampsia or eclampsia requires magnesium sulfate for seizure prevention and antihypertensives for blood pressure control. Diuretics and fluid restriction are adjuncts but not primary treatment. Oxytocin is unrelated to this hypertensive crisis.
SubChapter: Cardiopulmonary & Thromboembolic Complications
Q446. Answer: A
Explanation: Persistent depression requires professional evaluation and possibly pharmacologic treatment. It does not resolve spontaneously like postpartum blues. Support and therapy improve recovery and infant bonding, while isolation may worsen symptoms.
SubChapter: Psychological & Neurologic Conditions
Q447. Answer: A

Explanation: Prolonged rupture of membranes allows ascending bacteria, and cesarean incision adds exposure risk. Planned cesarean before rupture carries lower risk. Simple vaginal births rarely cause uterine infection.
SubChapter: Infectious Conditions
Q448. Answer: A
Explanation: The hypothyroid phase of postpartum thyroiditis appears months after birth with fatigue, weight gain, and dry skin. Cushing's involves hypercortisolism and muscle wasting; Addison's presents with hypotension and hyperpigmentation; diabetes shows polyuria and hyperglycemia.
SubChapter: Metabolic & Endocrine Disorders
Q449. Answer: C
Explanation: Development of a localized abscess requires incision and drainage plus continued antibiotics. Warm compresses alone are inadequate, and breastfeeding may continue from the unaffected breast. Stopping lactation increases engorgement risk.
SubChapter: Infectious Conditions
Q450. Answer: B
Explanation: Methylergonovine can cause dangerous vasoconstriction and hypertension; immediate discontinuation and provider notification are required. Further doses risk stroke or seizure. These symptoms are not expected effects.
SubChapter: Hematologic & Hemorrhagic Disorders
Q451. Answer: B
Explanation: Sudden dyspnea and hypoxia suggest pulmonary embolism. Elevating the head eases breathing, and oxygen improves saturation while awaiting emergency care. Flat positioning and exertion worsen hypoxia. Methylergonovine is unrelated to embolic management.
SubChapter: Cardiopulmonary & Thromboembolic Complications
Q452. Answer: A
Explanation: These findings indicate endometritis, a uterine infection requiring prompt antibiotic therapy. Fluids and comfort measures support recovery but are secondary. Delaying treatment increases the risk of septicemia.
SubChapter: Infectious Conditions
Q453. Answer: B
Explanation: Methylergonovine causes vasoconstriction and is contraindicated in hypertension due to stroke risk. Diabetes, asthma, and parity do not preclude its use but require routine monitoring.
SubChapter: Hematologic & Hemorrhagic Disorders
Q454. Answer: A
Explanation: Auditory hallucinations indicate postpartum psychosis, a psychiatric emergency requiring immediate intervention for maternal and infant safety. Support or rest alone is insufficient and delays lifesaving treatment.
SubChapter: Psychological & Neurologic Conditions
Q455. Answer: B
Explanation: Iron replacement restores hemoglobin following blood loss once bleeding is controlled. Oxytocin and methylergonovine treat active hemorrhage, not anemia; magnesium sulfate prevents seizures in preeclampsia, not blood loss effects.
SubChapter: Hematologic & Hemorrhagic Disorders
Q456. Answer: C
Explanation: Wound separation and drainage confirm dehiscence, often due to infection or poor healing. Mild tenderness and low-grade fever are expected. Hematomas cause bruising without incision separation.
SubChapter: Infectious Conditions

Q457. Answer: A
Explanation: Postpartum eclampsia presents with seizures from persistent hypertension and endothelial dysfunction. Hypoglycemia causes altered consciousness, not tonic-clonic activity. Psychosis produces hallucinations, not seizures.
SubChapter: Cardiopulmonary & Thromboembolic Complications
Q458. Answer: B
Explanation: Doppler ultrasound confirms venous thrombosis by detecting impaired venous flow. Chest X-ray and ECG assess pulmonary or cardiac issues, while CBC provides non-specific findings.
SubChapter: Cardiopulmonary & Thromboembolic Complications
Q459. Answer: C
Explanation: Depression lasts beyond two weeks and includes guilt and hopelessness affecting daily function. Postpartum blues resolve quickly and improve with support. Fatigue alone is normal recovery.
SubChapter: Psychological & Neurologic Conditions
Q460. Answer: B
Explanation: Retained placental fragments cause late postpartum infection and bleeding; surgical evacuation and antibiotics are required. Oxytocin or iron alone will not eliminate infected tissue or prevent sepsis.
SubChapter: Infectious Conditions
Q461. Answer: B
Explanation: Pulmonary embolism results from migration of a deep vein thrombus, producing dyspnea, pleuritic pain, and hemoptysis. Pneumonia and atelectasis cause cough without leg swelling; heart failure presents with edema but not hemoptysis from embolic origin.
SubChapter: Cardiopulmonary & Thromboembolic Complications
Q462. Answer: B
Explanation: Persistent bleeding despite a firm uterus indicates trauma such as a vaginal or cervical laceration. Atony causes a boggy uterus; retained fragments cause delayed bleeding; DIC presents with generalized oozing, not localized bright bleeding.
SubChapter: Hematologic & Hemorrhagic Disorders
Q463. Answer: C
Explanation: Fever and localized induration indicate bacterial mastitis. Antibiotics and continued milk removal are necessary to prevent abscess formation. Ice packs and pumping alone do not treat infection, and discontinuing breastfeeding worsens engorgement.
SubChapter: Infectious Conditions
Q464. Answer: D
Explanation: Difficulty bonding and persistent sadness for more than two weeks indicate postpartum depression. Blues are transient, resolving within 14 days. Sleep and appetite changes occur in both but resolve more quickly in normal adjustment.
SubChapter: Psychological & Neurologic Conditions
Q465. Answer: B
Explanation: Anemia from blood loss causes pallor, weakness, and syncope. Pulmonary embolism presents with dyspnea; endometritis with fever; preeclampsia with hypertension. Iron therapy and nutrition are mainstays of treatment.
SubChapter: Hematologic & Hemorrhagic Disorders
Q466. Answer: B
Explanation: Pyelonephritis involves upper urinary tract infection with systemic fever and flank tenderness. Cystitis is limited to the bladder and lacks systemic signs. Endometritis affects the uterus, and pelvic abscess presents with localized pelvic pain, not urinary symptoms.
SubChapter: Infectious Conditions

Q467. Answer: B
Explanation: Postpartum OCD features intrusive thoughts and compulsive avoidance behaviors with preserved insight. Psychosis involves loss of reality; depression shows hopelessness; panic disorder has episodic autonomic symptoms unrelated to infant safety.
SubChapter: Psychological & Neurologic Conditions
Q468. Answer: D
Explanation: Wound infection requires culture and prompt provider notification for antibiotic therapy. Covering alone does not address infection, and heat may worsen inflammation. Observation delays care and risks deeper involvement.
SubChapter: Infectious Conditions
Q469. Answer: B
Explanation: Calf tenderness or a positive Homan's sign indicates venous thrombosis and requires further evaluation. Bilateral edema is common; coolness and absent pulses suggest arterial disease rather than venous.
SubChapter: Cardiopulmonary & Thromboembolic Complications
Q470. Answer: B
Explanation: Signs of infection at the episiotomy site require antibiotics and local wound management. Sitz baths provide comfort but do not eradicate infection. Observation or topical cream alone delays healing and increases systemic risk.
SubChapter: Infectious Conditions
Q471. Answer: A
Explanation: E. coli is the most common cause of endometritis following prolonged rupture of membranes due to ascending contamination. S. aureus usually causes wound or breast infections; Chlamydia produces chronic endometritis; Pseudomonas is uncommon postpartum.
SubChapter: Infectious Conditions
Q472. Answer: C
Explanation: These symptoms indicate thrombophlebitis; the leg should remain immobile to prevent embolization. Ambulation or massage can dislodge the clot. Compression therapy is inappropriate until diagnosis confirmation.
SubChapter: Cardiopulmonary & Thromboembolic Complications
Q473. Answer: B
Explanation: Iron therapy and diet rich in iron restore hemoglobin following blood loss. Hydration aids circulation but does not correct anemia. Complete bed rest is unnecessary unless symptomatic; oxytocin treats uterine atony, not anemia.
SubChapter: Hematologic & Hemorrhagic Disorders
Q474. Answer: B
Explanation: Postpartum preeclampsia presents within six weeks after birth and can progress to eclampsia if untreated. Symptoms include headache and visual changes with hypertension. Thyroiditis and depression lack hypertensive findings; hypoglycemia causes shakiness, not vision problems.
SubChapter: Cardiopulmonary & Thromboembolic Complications
Q475. Answer: B
Explanation: Persistence beyond two weeks indicates postpartum depression, requiring psychological assessment and support. Delaying evaluation risks worsening depression and impaired bonding. Rest and reassurance alone are inadequate.
SubChapter: Psychological & Neurologic Conditions
Q476. Answer: B

Explanation: Ongoing bleeding despite a firm uterus indicates retained tissue preventing uterine vessel closure. Infection causes odor and fever later, while hematoma leads to localized swelling, not continuous bleeding.
SubChapter: Hematologic & Hemorrhagic Disorders
Q477. Answer: A
Explanation: Development of a fluctuant mass signifies abscess formation requiring drainage plus antibiotics. Ice reduces pain but not infection, and breastfeeding can continue from the unaffected side.
SubChapter: Infectious Conditions
Q478. Answer: B
Explanation: Persistent hyperglycemia postpartum indicates overt diabetes rather than transient gestational changes. Hypoglycemia presents with tremors and confusion; thyroiditis causes fatigue without high glucose; anemia results in pallor, not polydipsia.
SubChapter: Metabolic & Endocrine Disorders
Q479. Answer: C
Explanation: Postpartum depression persists beyond two weeks and disrupts normal functioning. Baby blues resolve within days. Recognizing duration and impairment guides timely mental health referral.
SubChapter: Psychological & Neurologic Conditions
Q480. Answer: B
Explanation: These findings reflect postpartum preeclampsia, which can progress to eclampsia with seizures if untreated. Magnesium sulfate prevents convulsions. Sepsis and embolism show different patterns; DIC is secondary to hemorrhage, not hypertension.
SubChapter: Cardiopulmonary & Thromboembolic Complications
Q481. Answer: B
Explanation: Postpartum cardiomyopathy is a form of heart failure occurring within months of delivery, characterized by pulmonary congestion and dyspnea. Pulmonary embolism is sudden with pleuritic pain; pneumonia causes fever; amniotic fluid embolism occurs intrapartum, not days later.
SubChapter: Cardiopulmonary & Thromboembolic Complications
Q482. Answer: C
Explanation: Elevated WBC with left shift confirms bacterial infection, consistent with endometritis. A firm, non-tender uterus suggests normal involution. Hydration alone doesn't normalize fever in infection.
SubChapter: Infectious Conditions
Q483. Answer: C
Explanation: Persistent sadness, apathy, and loss of functioning indicate postpartum depression. Hallucinations signal psychosis; mood swings with recovery represent blues; fatigue alone reflects physical adjustment.
SubChapter: Psychological & Neurologic Conditions
Q484. Answer: B
Explanation: Retained placental fragments maintain blood flow despite a firm uterus, causing delayed bleeding. Atony results in a boggy uterus; infection causes odor and fever; hematoma presents with localized swelling and pain.
SubChapter: Hematologic & Hemorrhagic Disorders
Q485. Answer: A
Explanation: Suspected DVT requires leg elevation and immobility to prevent clot migration. Massage or ambulation risks embolization; compression stockings are contraindicated until diagnosis is confirmed.
SubChapter: Cardiopulmonary & Thromboembolic Complications
Q486. Answer: A

Explanation: Postpartum blues occur within the first two weeks due to hormonal shifts and resolve spontaneously. Depression persists longer with impaired functioning, while psychosis presents with delusions or hallucinations.
SubChapter: Psychological & Neurologic Conditions

Q487. Answer: B

Explanation: Rapid fluid administration may cause pulmonary edema and fluid overload, indicated by crackles and JVD. Pulmonary embolism shows chest pain and hypoxia without rales; pneumonia includes fever; endometritis affects the uterus.
SubChapter: Cardiopulmonary & Thromboembolic Complications

Q488. Answer: A

Explanation: Hyperthyroid phase of postpartum thyroiditis causes tremors, anxiety, tachycardia, and weight loss. Later, fatigue and weight gain develop during hypothyroid phase. Other symptoms listed are unrelated to thyroid dysfunction.
SubChapter: Metabolic & Endocrine Disorders

Q489. Answer: B

Explanation: Continued milk removal through feeding or pumping prevents milk stasis and aids healing. Stopping feeds increases engorgement and worsens infection. Cold compresses alone are insufficient, and avoiding drainage prolongs inflammation.
SubChapter: Infectious Conditions

Q490. Answer: B

Explanation: A tense, purple, and painful swelling indicates a hematoma from vessel rupture. Infection shows erythema and drainage; lacerations cause visible bleeding; normal healing involves mild discomfort without swelling.
SubChapter: Hematologic & Hemorrhagic Disorders

Q491. Answer: B

Explanation: A firm uterus with persistent bleeding suggests retained placental fragments that prevent full vascular closure. Atony causes a soft uterus; infection causes fever; lacerations present immediately postpartum, not a week later.
SubChapter: Hematologic & Hemorrhagic Disorders

Q492. Answer: B

Explanation: Pulmonary embolism presents abruptly with chest pain, tachypnea, and dyspnea. Crackles and frothy sputum indicate heart failure; fever and cough point to pneumonia; bradycardia rarely occurs in embolism.
SubChapter: Cardiopulmonary & Thromboembolic Complications

Q493. Answer: A

Explanation: Symptoms lasting beyond two weeks indicate postpartum depression requiring professional evaluation. Early treatment prevents deterioration. Rest alone is insufficient, and reassurance delays needed intervention.
SubChapter: Psychological & Neurologic Conditions

Q494. Answer: B

Explanation: Wound infection with purulent drainage requires immediate culture and provider notification for antibiotics. Ice and ambulation delay appropriate treatment, and routine care alone cannot manage infection.
SubChapter: Infectious Conditions

Q495. Answer: B

Explanation: Magnesium sulfate prevents seizures in postpartum preeclampsia until blood pressure stabilizes. Oxytocin promotes uterine contraction, not seizure prevention. Terbutaline relaxes smooth muscle, and methylergonovine worsens hypertension.

SubChapter: Cardiopulmonary & Thromboembolic Complications

Q496. Answer: B

Explanation: Continuing breastfeeding and using warm compresses enhance milk drainage and healing in mastitis. Restricting flow worsens engorgement, and milk is safe if antibiotics are compatible.

SubChapter: Infectious Conditions

Q497. Answer: A

Explanation: The hypothyroid phase of postpartum thyroiditis develops several weeks after delivery, causing fatigue and weight gain. Diabetes and preeclampsia show metabolic and vascular changes, not cold intolerance. Depression lacks physical endocrine features.

SubChapter: Metabolic & Endocrine Disorders

Q498. Answer: B

Explanation: DIC follows obstetric complications like retained placenta, leading to widespread clotting factor consumption and diffuse bleeding. Anemia and embolism do not cause oozing, and endometritis presents with fever, not bleeding from multiple sites.

SubChapter: Hematologic & Hemorrhagic Disorders

Q499. Answer: B

Explanation: Postpartum psychosis is a psychiatric emergency requiring immediate provider notification and safety precautions. Supportive measures alone are inadequate. Delay increases risk of harm to mother and infant.

SubChapter: Psychological & Neurologic Conditions

Q500. Answer: A

Explanation: Cystitis requires antibiotics and hydration to eliminate infection and prevent spread. Restricting fluids or delaying therapy risks progression to pyelonephritis. Comfort measures alone are insufficient.

SubChapter: Infectious Conditions

Questions (501-600)

Q501. A woman presents with fever, lower abdominal pain, and foul-smelling lochia three days postpartum. Which is the best initial nursing intervention?

A. Encourage ambulation

B. Notify provider and prepare for antibiotic therapy

C. Apply ice to abdomen

D. Increase fluid intake only

Q502. Which postpartum condition is characterized by persistent bleeding despite a firm uterus and no visible laceration?

A. Retained placental fragments

B. Uterine atony

C. DIC

D. Endometritis

Q503. A woman develops calf pain, swelling, and warmth one week after cesarean delivery. Which diagnostic test confirms the suspected condition?

A. Venous Doppler ultrasound

B. Chest X-ray

C. ECG

D. Arterial blood gas

Q504. A postpartum patient reports sadness, lack of motivation, and fatigue for three weeks. Which nursing statement is appropriate?

A. "These feelings are normal and will pass soon."

B. "You may be experiencing postpartum depression; professional help can support recovery."

C. "Try resting more and increase fluids."

D. "Avoid discussing your feelings until hormones stabilize."

Q505. Which finding differentiates mastitis from a blocked milk duct?

A. Localized breast tenderness only

B. Absence of systemic symptoms

C. Fever and malaise accompanying breast pain

D. Pain relieved by feeding

Q506. A patient who experienced postpartum hemorrhage now exhibits oozing from gums and IV sites. Laboratory tests reveal low fibrinogen. Which disorder is suspected?

A. Anemia

B. DIC

C. Hypocalcemia

D. Endometritis

Q507. A postpartum client reports chest tightness, tachycardia, and shortness of breath three days after cesarean birth. What should the nurse do first?

A. Administer oxygen and elevate the head of the bed

B. Encourage coughing and deep breathing

C. Provide fluids for hydration

D. Massage lower extremities

Q508. A woman experiences tremor, anxiety, and weight loss six weeks postpartum. Which lab test best confirms the suspected diagnosis?

A. Thyroid-stimulating hormone (TSH)

B. Fasting glucose

C. Hemoglobin and hematocrit

D. Serum cortisol

Q509. A woman presents with high fever, uterine tenderness, and chills five days after delivery. Which factor most likely contributed to this condition?

A. Elective cesarean section
B. Prolonged rupture of membranes before birth
C. Rapid labor
D. Short second stage

Q510. A postpartum patient reports mood elevation followed by irritability and insomnia. She speaks rapidly and engages in impulsive spending. What condition is suspected?

A. Postpartum depression
B. Postpartum psychosis with manic features
C. Postpartum blues
D. Generalized anxiety

Q511. A postpartum client reports persistent perineal pain and pressure. The nurse notes a swollen, bluish area near the vaginal opening. What complication should be suspected?

A. Vaginal hematoma
B. Laceration infection
C. Uterine atony
D. Retained placenta

Q512. A woman presents four days postpartum with severe headache, blurred vision, and BP 168/108 mm Hg. Which medication should be administered first?

A. Magnesium sulfate
B. Oxytocin
C. Furosemide
D. Methylergonovine

Q513. A postpartum patient develops tachycardia, dyspnea, and low oxygen saturation two days after cesarean section. Which finding supports pulmonary embolism?

A. Bradycardia
B. Crackles and productive cough
C. Sudden chest pain and anxiety
D. Fever and chills

Q514. A postpartum client reports feelings of guilt, inability to sleep, and disinterest in her baby for one month. What is the best response by the nurse?

A. "These feelings are normal and will pass soon."
B. "You may have postpartum depression; let's discuss a referral for help."
C. "Try to rest more when the baby sleeps."
D. "Focus on caring for your baby to improve your mood."

Q515. A woman with postpartum hemorrhage continues bleeding despite oxytocin and uterine massage. Which second-line uterotonic is contraindicated in hypertension?

A. Carboprost tromethamine
B. Methylergonovine
C. Misoprostol
D. Tranexamic acid

Q516. A postpartum patient with mastitis asks if she can continue breastfeeding. What is the correct nursing response?

A. "You should stop breastfeeding until the infection clears."
B. "Continue breastfeeding or pumping to promote drainage."
C. "Breastfeed only on the unaffected side."

D. "Avoid expressing milk to prevent irritation."

Q517. A woman reports anxiety, obsessive thoughts about her infant's safety, and repetitive checking behaviors but recognizes they are excessive. Which diagnosis is most consistent?

A. Postpartum depression
B. Anxiety neurosis
C. Postpartum psychosis
D. Postpartum obsessive–compulsive disorder

Q518. A postpartum client develops fever, chills, and tenderness over the breast with localized redness. Which organism most commonly causes this infection?

A. Escherichia coli
B. Staphylococcus aureus
C. Klebsiella pneumoniae
D. Streptococcus pyogenes

Q519. A woman reports persistent fatigue, dry skin, and weight gain six months postpartum. What is the most likely cause?

A. Postpartum thyroiditis – hypothyroid phase
B. Diabetes mellitus
C. Adrenal insufficiency
D. Iron deficiency anemia

Q520. A patient develops confusion and agitation three days postpartum, stating she hears voices telling her to harm herself. What is the nurse's first action?

A. Encourage rest and hydration
B. Notify the provider immediately and ensure safety
C. Reassure that hormonal changes cause mood swings
D. Encourage family to provide support at home

Q521. A postpartum woman complains of severe headache, visual disturbances, and blood pressure of 170/110 mm Hg. What serious complication is she at risk for?

A. Pulmonary embolism
B. Eclampsia
C. DIC
D. Endometritis

Q522. A patient develops bright-red bleeding 12 days after delivery, and ultrasound shows retained placental fragments. Which treatment should the nurse anticipate?

A. Iron supplementation
B. Dilation and curettage
C. Oxytocin infusion only
D. Expectant management

Q523. A postpartum client reports shortness of breath and chest pain with an SpO_2 of 85%. What is the immediate nursing priority?

A. Administer oxygen and elevate the head of the bed
B. Encourage coughing and deep breathing
C. Provide fluids and observe
D. Massage calves for comfort

Q524. A woman describes feeling persistently sad and worthless one month after giving birth, expressing guilt about her inability to bond with her baby. What is the most likely diagnosis?

A. Postpartum blues
B. Postpartum depression
C. Postpartum psychosis

D. Generalized anxiety disorder

Q525. A postpartum client complains of fever, malaise, and localized breast pain that worsens during feeding. Which measure best supports recovery?

A. Stop breastfeeding temporarily

B. Continue breastfeeding and apply warm compresses

C. Apply cold compresses only

D. Wear a tight bra for support

Q526. A woman experiences sudden confusion and seizures five days after birth. She was previously diagnosed with mild hypertension. What is the likely diagnosis?

A. Eclampsia

B. Postpartum thyroiditis

C. Pulmonary embolism

D. Hypoglycemia

Q527. A patient who received multiple blood transfusions after hemorrhage now shows petechiae, oozing, and prolonged PT/aPTT. Which complication is suspected?

A. DIC

B. Sepsis

C. Anemia

D. Thrombophlebitis

Q528. Which postpartum symptom most clearly indicates hypothyroidism?

A. Tremors, sweating, and tachycardia

B. Fatigue, constipation, and cold intolerance

C. Anxiety and palpitations

D. Fever and chills

Q529. A woman one week postpartum reports persistent intrusive thoughts about accidentally harming her baby, though she recognizes them as irrational. What is the appropriate response?

A. Provide reassurance and suggest rest

B. Notify provider for evaluation of postpartum OCD

C. Encourage family support only

D. Suggest suppressing such thoughts

Q530. A postpartum client has persistent fever, uterine tenderness, and malodorous lochia after prolonged rupture of membranes. Which factor most likely contributed to this infection?

A. Short second stage

B. Prolonged labor and membrane rupture

C. Multiparity

D. Rapid vaginal birth

Q531. A postpartum woman presents with temperature 102°F, uterine tenderness, and foul-smelling lochia on day five after delivery. What is the likely diagnosis?

A. Endometritis

B. Cystitis

C. Mastitis

D. Wound infection

Q532. A postpartum client with severe hemorrhage develops oozing from venipuncture sites and gums. Laboratory tests reveal low fibrinogen and prolonged clotting times. Which is the correct interpretation?

A. Iron deficiency anemia

B. Disseminated intravascular coagulation

C. Hypocalcemia

D. Sepsis

Q533. A postpartum woman experiences chest pain, shortness of breath, and tachycardia. Oxygen saturation is 82%. Which intervention should be performed first?

A. Place patient in high Fowler's position and administer oxygen
B. Give diuretics to reduce fluid overload
C. Encourage ambulation
D. Administer methylergonovine

Q534. A woman reports feeling detached from reality and hearing voices telling her to harm her newborn two days after delivery. What should the nurse do first?

A. Notify the provider and ensure constant supervision
B. Provide reassurance that mood changes are common
C. Encourage rest and relaxation techniques
D. Offer supportive counseling and discharge education

Q535. A woman who delivered by cesarean complains of pain, redness, and swelling at the incision site with purulent drainage. What is the most appropriate action?

A. Apply a clean dry dressing and monitor
B. Obtain wound culture and notify provider
C. Reassure this is part of healing
D. Apply cold compresses only

Q536. A postpartum patient reports extreme fatigue and pallor two weeks after a significant hemorrhage. Which laboratory test best evaluates her condition?

A. Complete blood count
B. Urinalysis
C. Coagulation profile
D. Blood glucose

Q537. A woman reports persistent sadness and hopelessness for four weeks after delivery, along with loss of appetite. What is the likely diagnosis?

A. Postpartum blues
B. Postpartum depression
C. Postpartum psychosis
D. Anxiety disorder

Q538. A nurse assessing a woman 12 days postpartum notes heavy bleeding with a firm uterus and normal vital signs. What is the most probable cause?

A. Retained placental fragments
B. Uterine atony
C. Endometritis
D. Vaginal laceration

Q539. A patient presents with heat intolerance, tachycardia, and weight loss six weeks postpartum. Which laboratory result would support the diagnosis?

A. Low TSH and elevated free T_4
B. Elevated TSH and low free T_4
C. Normal TSH and T_4
D. Elevated TSH and normal T_4

Q540. A woman who had a prolonged labor and cesarean birth develops high fever, tachycardia, and foul uterine discharge. What is the most likely cause?

A. Endometritis
B. DIC
C. Preeclampsia

D. Mastitis

Q541. A woman experiences shortness of breath, chest pain, and tachycardia five days after a cesarean birth. Which assessment finding would confirm pulmonary embolism?

A. Slow shallow respirations
B. Low blood pressure with bradycardia
C. Crackles throughout both lungs
D. Sudden drop in oxygen saturation

Q542. A postpartum client reports fever, uterine tenderness, and foul-smelling lochia three days after delivery. What is the most important nursing action?

A. Administer prescribed antibiotics and monitor vital signs
B. Encourage ambulation to promote uterine drainage
C. Apply an ice pack to reduce tenderness
D. Increase fluid intake only

Q543. A woman with postpartum hemorrhage shows petechiae, oozing at IV sites, and prolonged clotting times. What diagnosis is most consistent?

A. DIC
B. Preeclampsia
C. Anemia
D. Thrombophlebitis

Q544. A postpartum woman complains of severe headache and blurred vision, and her BP is 165/105 mm Hg. Which intervention should be initiated?

A. Administer magnesium sulfate and antihypertensive medication
B. Provide oral fluids
C. Encourage rest and deep breathing
D. Apply cold compresses to the head

Q545. A patient reports sadness, fatigue, and loss of interest in her newborn persisting for over a month. What is the best nursing intervention?

A. Suggest waiting a few more weeks
B. Advise more rest and fluids
C. Encourage psychiatric evaluation and supportive counseling
D. Reassure that the mood swings are temporary

Q546. A woman reports breast tenderness, fever, and a localized painful lump. She is on antibiotics for mastitis but now has purulent drainage. Which complication developed?

A. Breast abscess
B. Blocked milk duct
C. Engorgement
D. Cystitis

Q547. A woman with severe postpartum hemorrhage shows hypotension, tachycardia, and pale, cool skin. Which nursing priority is correct?

A. Begin fluid resuscitation and notify provider
B. Encourage oral hydration
C. Elevate legs and reassess in one hour
D. Apply ice to abdomen

Q548. A patient develops fever and chills five days postpartum after prolonged rupture of membranes. What teaching should the nurse provide?

A. Complete the full course of prescribed antibiotics
B. Ambulate to encourage drainage
C. Avoid breastfeeding until fever subsides

D. Apply perineal ice packs hourly

Q549. A woman presents with fatigue, cold intolerance, and weight gain four months postpartum. What finding supports the suspected diagnosis?

A. Normal thyroid profile

B. Low TSH and high free T_4

C. Elevated TSH and low free T_4

D. Elevated free T_4 with normal TSH

Q550. A postpartum patient becomes anxious, restless, and reports hearing voices instructing her to harm her baby. What is the immediate nursing priority?

A. Maintain safety and notify the provider immediately

B. Provide reassurance and quiet environment

C. Offer sleep medication

D. Encourage deep breathing exercises

Q551. A postpartum woman develops heavy vaginal bleeding one week after delivery with a firm, midline uterus. Which cause is most likely?

A. Retained placental fragments

B. Uterine atony

C. Cervical tear

D. DIC

Q552. A patient develops fever, tachycardia, and uterine tenderness three days postpartum. Lochia is foul smelling. Which infection is suspected?

A. Endometritis

B. Mastitis

C. Urinary tract infection

D. Wound infection

Q553. A woman experiences severe dyspnea, hypotension, and cyanosis immediately after birth. What is the likely cause?

A. Heart failure

B. Pulmonary embolism

C. Pneumonia

D. Amniotic fluid embolism

Q554. A postpartum client reports persistent feelings of worthlessness and inability to care for her baby for five weeks. Which action should the nurse take?

A. Refer to a mental health provider immediately

B. Reassure her symptoms will resolve naturally

C. Suggest relaxation exercises

D. Recommend temporary separation from infant

Q555. A woman with postpartum hemorrhage fails to respond to oxytocin. Methylergonovine is ordered, but her BP is 170/100 mm Hg. What should the nurse do?

A. Hold the medication and notify provider

B. Administer as ordered with monitoring

C. Give an IV bolus for rapid action

D. Substitute with misoprostol

Q556. A postpartum woman presents with breast pain, redness, and a palpable fluctuant area despite antibiotic therapy. What intervention is expected?

A. Incision and drainage of abscess

B. Continue antibiotics only

C. Apply ice packs and tight bra

D. Stop breastfeeding permanently

Q557. A patient develops seizures five days postpartum following elevated BP and headache. Which medication should be continued during stabilization?

A. Furosemide
B. Oxytocin
C. Magnesium sulfate
D. Methylergonovine

Q558. A woman reports restlessness, racing thoughts, decreased need for sleep, and excessive spending two weeks after birth. What condition should be suspected?

A. Postpartum psychosis with manic features
B. Postpartum blues
C. Generalized anxiety disorder
D. Depression

Q559. A woman with postpartum hemorrhage now exhibits oozing from gums and IV sites. Laboratory tests reveal low fibrinogen. Which disorder is suspected?

A. Postpartum thyroiditis – hyperthyroid phase
B. Postpartum depression
C. Hypocalcemia
D. Diabetes mellitus

Q560. A woman reports fever, flank pain, and dysuria 10 days after delivery. Urinalysis reveals bacteria and white blood cells. What is the correct management?

A. Start antibiotics and increase oral fluids
B. Encourage rest and observation only
C. Administer uterotonic medication
D. Restrict fluids to reduce frequency

Q561. A postpartum client develops shortness of breath, anxiety, and chest pain two days after cesarean section. Her oxygen saturation is 83%. What complication should the nurse suspect?

A. Pulmonary embolism
B. Pneumonia
C. Atelectasis
D. Heart failure

Q562. A woman reports persistent heavy bleeding and dizziness one week postpartum, with a firm, midline uterus. What is the most probable cause?

A. DIC
B. Uterine atony
C. Retained placental fragments
D. Perineal hematoma

Q563. A postpartum client complains of fever, uterine tenderness, and foul-smelling lochia four days after delivery. What is the correct nursing action?

A. Notify provider and prepare to start IV antibiotics
B. Encourage ambulation and fluids
C. Provide reassurance and monitor temperature
D. Apply ice to the abdomen

Q564. A postpartum woman develops blurred vision, severe headache, and blood pressure 168/108 mm Hg on day five. What medication should be prioritized?

A. Magnesium sulfate
B. Methylergonovine
C. Oxytocin

D. Furosemide

Q565. A woman complains of sadness, fatigue, and inability to enjoy her baby for four weeks after delivery. What should the nurse recommend?

A. Immediate mental health referral for postpartum depression
B. Rest and hydration only
C. Reassurance that hormones will normalize
D. Isolation from visitors to reduce stress

Q566. A woman who had postpartum hemorrhage now exhibits oozing from venipuncture sites, low fibrinogen, and prolonged clotting times. Which diagnosis fits best?

A. Thrombophlebitis
B. Anemia
C. Endometritis
D. DIC

Q567. A postpartum client develops high fever, red streaks on the breast, and malaise while breastfeeding. Which nursing advice is correct?

A. Continue breastfeeding and apply warm compresses
B. Stop breastfeeding immediately
C. Wear a tight bra for support
D. Express milk and discard it

Q568. A patient reports anxiety, racing thoughts, and excessive energy two weeks postpartum. She sleeps less but denies sadness. What condition is likely?

A. Postpartum psychosis with manic features
B. Postpartum depression
C. Anxiety disorder
D. Postpartum blues

Q569. A woman six months postpartum reports fatigue, weight gain, constipation, and cold intolerance. Which lab pattern supports the suspected diagnosis?

A. Elevated TSH, low T_4
B. Low TSH, high T_4
C. Normal TSH and T_4
D. Elevated cortisol

Q570. A postpartum woman becomes acutely confused and agitated, stating she hears voices commanding her to harm her baby. What is the nurse's first priority?

A. Encourage rest and fluids
B. Reassure her that this is temporary
C. Ensure safety and notify the provider immediately
D. Provide family teaching about mood swings

Q571. A 36-week neonate presents with grunting, nasal flaring, and intercostal retractions shortly after birth. Chest x-ray shows a ground-glass appearance. Which diagnosis is most likely?

A. Meconium aspiration syndrome
B. Transient tachypnea of the newborn
C. Respiratory distress syndrome
D. Persistent pulmonary hypertension

Q572. A term newborn with cyanosis and tachypnea improves when crying but worsens while feeding. Which defect is most consistent?

A. Choanal atresia
B. Coarctation of the aorta
C. Tetralogy of Fallot

D. Pulmonary hypoplasia

Q573. A newborn with Down syndrome develops persistent vomiting and an abdominal "double-bubble" sign on x-ray. What is the likely diagnosis?

A. Duodenal atresia
B. Pyloric stenosis
C. Hirschsprung disease
D. Meconium ileus

Q574. A neonate presents with anemia, jaundice, and elevated reticulocyte count on day 2 of life. Direct antiglobulin test is positive. What is the most likely cause?

A. Glucose-6-phosphate dehydrogenase deficiency
B. Rh hemolytic disease
C. ABO incompatibility with type O mother
D. Physiologic jaundice

Q575. A preterm infant (30 weeks) develops abdominal distention, bloody stools, and pneumatosis intestinalis on imaging. Which management step is most urgent?

A. Start enteral feeds
B. Surgical resection
C. Stop feeds and begin broad-spectrum antibiotics
D. Administer proton pump inhibitor

Q576. A term infant presents with lethargy, jitteriness, and blood glucose < 30 mg/dL after birth to a diabetic mother. What is the most appropriate initial treatment?

A. Oral sucrose drops
B. IV dextrose bolus followed by infusion
C. Feed formula and recheck in 2 hours
D. Glucagon IM only

Q577. A newborn with poor feeding and umbilical stump erythema develops temperature instability and hypotonia. What should be done first?

A. Observe and repeat vitals
B. Draw cultures and start IV antibiotics
C. Administer acetaminophen
D. Delay evaluation until fever develops

Q578. A neonate with persistent hypoxia and loud single S2 on exam is diagnosed with transposition of the great arteries (TGA). Which initial therapy stabilizes oxygenation before surgery?

A. IV furosemide
B. Prostaglandin E1 infusion
C. Phenylephrine infusion
D. Beta-blocker therapy

Q579. A preterm infant develops recurrent apnea and bradycardia spells during sleep. Which medication is indicated to reduce these episodes?

A. Morphine
B. Caffeine citrate
C. Lorazepam
D. Phenobarbital

Q580. A 2-day-old neonate becomes lethargic with poor perfusion and metabolic acidosis. Echocardiogram shows a patent ductus arteriosus-dependent systemic circulation. Which congenital defect is consistent?

A. Coarctation of the aorta
B. Ventricular septal defect

C. Atrial septal defect
D. Pulmonary stenosis

Q581. A 3-day-old term infant develops jaundice, lethargy, and poor feeding. Total bilirubin is 26 mg/dL. What complication is most concerning if untreated?
A. Kernicterus
B. Anemia
C. Sepsis
D. Dehydration

Q582. A 34-week premature infant develops apnea, temperature instability, and abdominal distention. Blood culture grows E. coli. What maternal factor most likely contributed?
A. Oligohydramnios
B. Prolonged rupture of membranes
C. Placenta previa
D. Preeclampsia

Q583. A newborn has a high-pitched cry, tremors, sneezing, and diarrhea within 48 hours of birth. The mother was on methadone therapy. What is the diagnosis?
A. Hypocalcemia
B. Neonatal abstinence syndrome
C. Sepsis
D. Intracranial hemorrhage

Q584. A term infant has tachypnea, hepatomegaly, and a holosystolic murmur at the lower left sternal border. What is the most probable diagnosis?
A. Ventricular septal defect
B. Patent ductus arteriosus
C. Aortic stenosis
D. Coarctation of the aorta

Q585. A newborn exposed to poorly controlled maternal diabetes presents with macrosomia and respiratory distress. Chest x-ray shows low lung volumes and fine reticulogranular pattern. Primary cause?
A. Meconium aspiration
B. Surfactant deficiency
C. Pulmonary hypoplasia
D. Transient tachypnea

Q586. A neonate shows abdominal distention, failure to pass meconium, and explosive stool after rectal exam. What is the most likely diagnosis?
A. Meconium plug syndrome
B. Hirschsprung disease
C. Cystic fibrosis
D. Anal stenosis

Q587. A neonate has microcephaly, cataracts, and a continuous murmur. Maternal records show rash during early pregnancy. Which infection is most likely?
A. Toxoplasmosis
B. Rubella
C. Cytomegalovirus
D. Syphilis

Q588. A 2-day-old term infant presents with seizures, hypocalcemia, and hypomagnesemia. Mother has poorly controlled diabetes. Most likely explanation?
A. Birth trauma

B. Maternal hyperparathyroidism
C. Delayed parathyroid hormone synthesis
D. Hypoxic-ischemic injury

Q589. A premature infant develops pallor, tachycardia, and low hematocrit without bleeding. Reticulocyte count is low. Which mechanism explains this anemia?
A. Hemolysis from maternal antibodies
B. Decreased erythropoietin production
C. Vitamin K deficiency
D. Iron overload

Q590. A newborn with ambiguous genitalia has hyponatremia, hyperkalemia, and hypotension. Which disorder is most likely?
A. Congenital adrenal hyperplasia
B. Androgen insensitivity syndrome
C. Turner syndrome
D. Klinefelter syndrome

Q591. A preterm infant (32 weeks) develops tachypnea and intercostal retractions. X-ray reveals patchy infiltrates and air bronchograms. What is the first-line treatment?
A. Inhaled nitric oxide
B. Continuous positive airway pressure (CPAP)
C. Intravenous diuretics
D. Antibiotic therapy

Q592. A term neonate suddenly becomes cyanotic during feeding and exhibits choking episodes relieved by crying. Which defect should be suspected?
A. Esophageal atresia with tracheoesophageal fistula
B. Coarctation of the aorta
C. Bronchopulmonary dysplasia
D. Pulmonary sequestration

Q593. A neonate has pallor, mild jaundice, and hematocrit 25% with elevated reticulocytes on day 3. No maternal antibody detected. What is the probable diagnosis?
A. Physiologic anemia of the newborn
B. Anemia of prematurity
C. Fetomaternal hemorrhage
D. G6PD deficiency

Q594. A 4-day-old infant shows lethargy, temperature instability, and bulging fontanelle. CSF reveals elevated protein and low glucose. Most likely pathogen?
A. Listeria monocytogenes
B. Escherichia coli
C. Group B Streptococcus
D. Enterovirus

Q595. A male newborn has hypotonia, poor feeding, and undescended testes. Chromosome analysis shows 47,XXY. Which hormone pattern is typical later in life?
A. Low FSH, Low LH
B. High FSH, High LH
C. High FSH, Low LH
D. Normal FSH, High LH

Q596. A preterm infant on ventilator develops oxygen saturation fluctuations and intermittent hypoxemia. Transillumination shows bright glow on right chest. Diagnosis?
A. Pneumonia

B. Pneumothorax
C. Atelectasis
D. Pleural effusion

Q597. A newborn has vomiting and green bilious staining of nasogastric aspirate within hours of birth. X-ray shows no gas in the distal intestine. What is the next step?

A. Start oral feeds slowly
B. Emergency surgical consult for malrotation with volvulus
C. Administer oral contrast study
D. Observe for 24 hours

Q598. A 2-day-old infant presents with petechiae and thrombocytopenia. Mother has idiopathic thrombocytopenic purpura (ITP). Mechanism of infant's condition?

A. Decreased platelet production
B. Maternal antibody-mediated platelet destruction
C. Genetic platelet defect
D. Viral infection

Q599. A preterm infant develops conjunctivitis with copious purulent discharge on day 2 of life. What is the likely organism?

A. Chlamydia trachomatis
B. Pseudomonas aeruginosa
C. Staphylococcus aureus
D. Neisseria gonorrhoeae

Q600. A neonate presents with ambiguous genitalia and elevated 17-hydroxyprogesterone on screening. Which electrolyte imbalance is expected?

A. Hypernatremia, hypokalemia
B. Hyponatremia, hyperkalemia
C. Hypercalcemia, alkalosis
D. Normal electrolytes

Answer key and Explanation (501-600)

Q501. Answer: B
Explanation: Fever, uterine tenderness, and malodorous lochia indicate endometritis requiring prompt antibiotic treatment. Supportive measures like fluids or ambulation do not treat infection and delay definitive care.
SubChapter: Infectious Conditions
Q502. Answer: A
Explanation: Retained placental tissue maintains open uterine sinuses, causing prolonged bleeding with a firm uterus. Atony causes a soft fundus; DIC presents with generalized oozing; infection involves fever and tenderness, not isolated bleeding.
SubChapter: Hematologic & Hemorrhagic Disorders
Q503. Answer: A
Explanation: Venous Doppler ultrasound identifies thrombus and impaired venous flow, confirming DVT. Chest X-ray and ECG assess pulmonary or cardiac causes, while ABG evaluates gas exchange but not venous obstruction.
SubChapter: Cardiopulmonary & Thromboembolic Complications
Q504. Answer: B
Explanation: Symptoms lasting beyond two weeks indicate postpartum depression requiring early mental health support. Dismissing or delaying care increases risk of worsening mood and impaired bonding.
SubChapter: Psychological & Neurologic Conditions
Q505. Answer: C
Explanation: Systemic symptoms such as fever and malaise accompany bacterial mastitis, while blocked ducts cause localized discomfort without infection. Continued feeding helps relieve both conditions but does not differentiate them.
SubChapter: Infectious Conditions
Q506. Answer: B
Explanation: Disseminated intravascular coagulation follows massive blood loss or placental complications, producing widespread coagulation failure and low fibrinogen. Anemia causes pallor without bleeding; hypocalcemia causes tetany; endometritis involves infection, not coagulopathy.
SubChapter: Hematologic & Hemorrhagic Disorders
Q507. Answer: A
Explanation: These signs indicate pulmonary embolism requiring immediate oxygen and positioning for optimal ventilation while notifying the provider. Massage risks dislodging more clots, and fluids do not address hypoxia.
SubChapter: Cardiopulmonary & Thromboembolic Complications
Q508. Answer: A
Explanation: Low TSH confirms hyperthyroid phase of postpartum thyroiditis. Fasting glucose screens for diabetes, hematocrit for anemia, and cortisol for adrenal disorders, none matching the described symptoms.
SubChapter: Metabolic & Endocrine Disorders
Q509. Answer: B
Explanation: Prolonged rupture of membranes allows bacterial ascent, predisposing to endometritis. Elective cesarean with intact membranes and short labors carry lower risk. Preventive antibiotics reduce incidence.
SubChapter: Infectious Conditions
Q510. Answer: B

Explanation: Manic behavior, pressured speech, and insomnia indicate a psychotic episode with bipolar features. Depression lacks euphoria; blues are transient; anxiety presents with worry rather than impulsivity.
SubChapter: Psychological & Neurologic Conditions

Q511. Answer: A

Explanation: A tense, bluish perineal swelling indicates hematoma formation from vessel injury during delivery. Infection presents later with erythema and fever, while uterine atony and retained placenta cause uterine bleeding, not localized swelling.
SubChapter: Hematologic & Hemorrhagic Disorders

Q512. Answer: A

Explanation: These symptoms indicate postpartum preeclampsia; magnesium sulfate prevents seizures. Methylergonovine is contraindicated due to hypertension. Oxytocin and furosemide do not address neurologic irritability.
SubChapter: Cardiopulmonary & Thromboembolic Complications

Q513. Answer: C

Explanation: Sudden chest pain, tachycardia, and anxiety are hallmark symptoms of pulmonary embolism. Crackles with cough suggest pneumonia; fever with chills indicates infection; bradycardia is not typical.
SubChapter: Cardiopulmonary & Thromboembolic Complications

Q514. Answer: B

Explanation: Duration over two weeks and loss of bonding signify postpartum depression requiring referral. Dismissing or minimizing symptoms delays effective intervention and worsens outcomes.
SubChapter: Psychological & Neurologic Conditions

Q515. Answer: B

Explanation: Methylergonovine elevates blood pressure and is contraindicated in hypertensive patients. Carboprost and misoprostol are safe alternatives, and tranexamic acid supports clot stability rather than uterine contraction.
SubChapter: Hematologic & Hemorrhagic Disorders

Q516. Answer: B

Explanation: Frequent feeding or pumping promotes drainage and recovery in mastitis. Ceasing feeding worsens milk stasis and infection risk. Most antibiotics are safe for nursing.
SubChapter: Infectious Conditions

Q517. Answer: D

Explanation: Postpartum OCD features intrusive thoughts with intact insight. Psychosis involves hallucinations or delusions; depression involves sadness and withdrawal; generalized anxiety lacks compulsive checking.
SubChapter: Psychological & Neurologic Conditions

Q518. Answer: B

Explanation: S. aureus is the leading cause of mastitis due to nipple trauma and milk stasis. E. coli commonly affects the urinary tract, while Klebsiella and Streptococcus are less frequent in breast infections.
SubChapter: Infectious Conditions

Q519. Answer: A

Explanation: The hypothyroid phase of postpartum thyroiditis presents with fatigue, cold intolerance, and weight gain months after delivery. Diabetes causes hyperglycemia; adrenal insufficiency causes hypotension; anemia causes pallor but not dry skin.
SubChapter: Metabolic & Endocrine Disorders

Q520. Answer: B

Explanation: Postpartum psychosis is a psychiatric emergency requiring immediate intervention and safety precautions. Support and reassurance are secondary to securing treatment and protecting mother and infant.
SubChapter: Psychological & Neurologic Conditions
Q521. Answer: B
Explanation: Uncontrolled hypertension with neurologic symptoms indicates postpartum preeclampsia progressing toward eclampsia, characterized by seizures if untreated. Pulmonary embolism causes dyspnea; DIC causes bleeding; endometritis involves fever and uterine tenderness.
SubChapter: Cardiopulmonary & Thromboembolic Complications
Q522. Answer: B
Explanation: Retained placental fragments require surgical evacuation to stop bleeding and prevent infection. Oxytocin contracts the uterus but cannot remove retained tissue. Iron therapy corrects anemia but not the cause.
SubChapter: Hematologic & Hemorrhagic Disorders
Q523. Answer: A
Explanation: Sudden hypoxia and chest pain suggest pulmonary embolism. Immediate oxygen administration and upright positioning optimize gas exchange. Coughing and massage can worsen embolization.
SubChapter: Cardiopulmonary & Thromboembolic Complications
Q524. Answer: B
Explanation: Duration beyond two weeks with guilt and impaired bonding indicates postpartum depression. Blues resolve quickly; psychosis features delusions; anxiety lacks pervasive sadness or guilt.
SubChapter: Psychological & Neurologic Conditions
Q525. Answer: B
Explanation: Continued milk removal with warm compresses helps treat mastitis by relieving stasis and infection. Stopping feeds or compression increases engorgement and worsens symptoms.
SubChapter: Infectious Conditions
Q526. Answer: A
Explanation: Postpartum eclampsia causes seizures due to cerebral edema and hypertension. Thyroiditis presents with metabolic symptoms, not seizures; embolism causes dyspnea; hypoglycemia results in tremors and confusion, not convulsions.
SubChapter: Cardiopulmonary & Thromboembolic Complications
Q527. Answer: A
Explanation: Disseminated intravascular coagulation results from consumption of clotting factors following massive transfusion or obstetric trauma, causing bleeding from multiple sites. Sepsis causes fever; anemia causes pallor; thrombophlebitis involves localized pain.
SubChapter: Hematologic & Hemorrhagic Disorders
Q528. Answer: B
Explanation: The hypothyroid phase of postpartum thyroiditis presents with fatigue, weight gain, constipation, and sensitivity to cold. The hyperthyroid phase features tremors and anxiety. Fever and chills suggest infection.
SubChapter: Metabolic & Endocrine Disorders
Q529. Answer: B
Explanation: Recurrent intrusive thoughts with awareness reflect postpartum obsessive–compulsive disorder, warranting mental health evaluation and therapy. Ignoring symptoms or reassurance alone delays treatment.
SubChapter: Psychological & Neurologic Conditions
Q530. Answer: B

Explanation: Extended rupture of membranes and prolonged labor facilitate ascending bacterial infection leading to endometritis. Short or rapid labors and multiparity alone do not cause infection.
SubChapter: Infectious Conditions

Q531. Answer: A

Explanation: Endometritis, a common uterine infection after delivery, presents with fever, uterine tenderness, and malodorous lochia. Cystitis affects the urinary tract, mastitis involves the breast, and wound infections are localized to the incision.
SubChapter: Infectious Conditions

Q532. Answer: B

Explanation: DIC involves consumption of clotting factors after massive hemorrhage or placental complications. It causes bleeding from multiple sites and prolonged PT/aPTT. Anemia lacks coagulation changes, and sepsis primarily shows fever.
SubChapter: Hematologic & Hemorrhagic Disorders

Q533. Answer: A

Explanation: Sudden respiratory distress postpartum suggests pulmonary embolism. Immediate oxygen administration and upright positioning optimize ventilation while awaiting emergency care. Other actions delay life-saving intervention.
SubChapter: Cardiopulmonary & Thromboembolic Complications

Q534. Answer: A

Explanation: Hallucinations and disorganized thoughts indicate postpartum psychosis, a psychiatric emergency requiring immediate provider notification and safety measures. Delay in treatment risks harm to mother and infant.
SubChapter: Psychological & Neurologic Conditions

Q535. Answer: B

Explanation: Signs of wound infection require culture to identify organisms and guide antibiotic therapy. Covering or cooling the wound delays diagnosis and increases risk of deeper infection.
SubChapter: Infectious Conditions

Q536. Answer: A

Explanation: A CBC assesses hemoglobin and hematocrit to confirm anemia following blood loss. Coagulation studies evaluate clotting, not red cell levels; urinalysis and glucose are unrelated to anemia.
SubChapter: Hematologic & Hemorrhagic Disorders

Q537. Answer: B

Explanation: Postpartum depression lasts longer than two weeks, often accompanied by appetite and sleep changes. Blues are transient; psychosis presents with hallucinations; anxiety lacks sustained sadness.
SubChapter: Psychological & Neurologic Conditions

Q538. Answer: A

Explanation: Continued bleeding with a firm uterus suggests retained placental tissue, preventing full uterine involution. Atony causes a soft uterus, and infection or laceration usually presents sooner.
SubChapter: Hematologic & Hemorrhagic Disorders

Q539. Answer: A

Explanation: Hyperthyroid phase of postpartum thyroiditis shows low TSH and elevated free T_4. Hypothyroidism produces the opposite pattern. Normal results exclude thyroid disease.
SubChapter: Metabolic & Endocrine Disorders

Q540. Answer: A

Explanation: Endometritis follows prolonged labor or cesarean delivery, with fever, tachycardia, and malodorous lochia due to uterine infection. DIC involves bleeding; preeclampsia causes hypertension; mastitis affects the breast.

SubChapter: Infectious Conditions

Q541. Answer: D

Explanation: Sudden hypoxia with chest pain and tachycardia is classic for pulmonary embolism. Crackles suggest heart failure; bradycardia and shallow respirations are not typical findings. Immediate oxygen and emergency care are required.

SubChapter: Cardiopulmonary & Thromboembolic Complications

Q542. Answer: A

Explanation: Endometritis requires antibiotic therapy and close monitoring for sepsis. Ambulation and fluids may help but are not primary treatments. Ice offers minimal relief for uterine infection.

SubChapter: Infectious Conditions

Q543. Answer: A

Explanation: Disseminated intravascular coagulation follows massive hemorrhage or obstetric complications, causing diffuse bleeding due to clotting factor consumption. Preeclampsia may trigger it but lacks these findings alone.

SubChapter: Hematologic & Hemorrhagic Disorders

Q544. Answer: A

Explanation: Elevated BP with neurologic symptoms indicates postpartum preeclampsia, requiring seizure prevention and blood pressure control. Comfort or hydration alone is inadequate and delays treatment.

SubChapter: Cardiopulmonary & Thromboembolic Complications

Q545. Answer: C

Explanation: Postpartum depression lasting more than two weeks requires professional mental health referral. Delay in treatment increases risk for self-harm or poor infant bonding.

SubChapter: Psychological & Neurologic Conditions

Q546. Answer: A

Explanation: A fluctuant, draining area following mastitis indicates abscess formation requiring drainage and continued antibiotics. Engorgement causes bilateral swelling; a blocked duct lacks drainage; cystitis affects the urinary tract.

SubChapter: Infectious Conditions

Q547. Answer: A

Explanation: Rapid IV fluid resuscitation prevents shock in postpartum hemorrhage. Oral fluids are insufficient, and delays increase risk of cardiovascular collapse.

SubChapter: Hematologic & Hemorrhagic Disorders

Q548. Answer: A

Explanation: Completing antibiotics ensures eradication of infection and prevents recurrence. Ambulation helps but does not treat infection; breastfeeding is safe unless contraindicated by medication.

SubChapter: Infectious Conditions

Q549. Answer: C

Explanation: Elevated TSH with low T_4 indicates hypothyroid phase of postpartum thyroiditis. Opposite findings suggest hyperthyroidism. Normal values exclude thyroid disease.

SubChapter: Metabolic & Endocrine Disorders

Q550. Answer: A

Explanation: Postpartum psychosis requires immediate safety precautions and urgent psychiatric care to prevent harm. Reassurance and relaxation are not substitutes for emergency intervention.

SubChapter: Psychological & Neurologic Conditions

Q551. Answer: A

Explanation: Retained placental fragments maintain blood flow despite uterine firmness. Atony causes a soft uterus; cervical tears bleed immediately postpartum; DIC involves diffuse oozing, not isolated uterine bleeding.
SubChapter: Hematologic & Hemorrhagic Disorders

Q552. Answer: A

Explanation: Endometritis presents with uterine tenderness, fever, and malodorous lochia due to infection of the endometrial lining. Mastitis and wound infection involve localized breast or incision pain, not uterine tenderness.
SubChapter: Infectious Conditions

Q553. Answer: D

Explanation: Amniotic fluid embolism occurs suddenly during or immediately after delivery, causing cardiovascular collapse and respiratory distress. Pulmonary embolism occurs later; pneumonia and heart failure develop gradually.
SubChapter: Cardiopulmonary & Thromboembolic Complications

Q554. Answer: A

Explanation: Prolonged depression with loss of function indicates postpartum depression requiring professional evaluation. Reassurance or avoidance strategies delay treatment and worsen outcomes.
SubChapter: Psychological & Neurologic Conditions

Q555. Answer: A

Explanation: Methylergonovine is contraindicated in hypertension due to risk of stroke. The nurse should withhold it and contact the provider. Misoprostol may be used instead.
SubChapter: Hematologic & Hemorrhagic Disorders

Q556. Answer: A

Explanation: Development of a fluctuant mass after mastitis indicates abscess formation requiring drainage. Breastfeeding may continue from the unaffected side. Ice or compression alone is inadequate.
SubChapter: Infectious Conditions

Q557. Answer: C

Explanation: Magnesium sulfate prevents and controls seizures in eclampsia. Oxytocin manages uterine tone, furosemide aids fluid removal, and methylergonovine is contraindicated in hypertension.
SubChapter: Cardiopulmonary & Thromboembolic Complications

Q558. Answer: A

Explanation: Manic symptoms following childbirth indicate bipolar-type postpartum psychosis. Depression lacks euphoria; blues resolve within two weeks; anxiety involves worry, not impulsivity or insomnia.
SubChapter: Psychological & Neurologic Conditions

Q559. Answer: A

Explanation: Hyperthyroid phase of postpartum thyroiditis produces adrenergic symptoms including tremors and anxiety. Depression affects mood, hypocalcemia causes muscle spasms, and diabetes leads to polyuria and hyperglycemia.
SubChapter: Metabolic & Endocrine Disorders

Q560. Answer: A

Explanation: Pyelonephritis presents with systemic fever and flank pain; treatment requires antibiotics and hydration to prevent sepsis. Uterotonics and fluid restriction are inappropriate.
SubChapter: Infectious Conditions

Q561. Answer: A

Explanation: Sudden dyspnea and hypoxia following cesarean delivery strongly suggest pulmonary embolism from venous thrombosis. It presents abruptly with chest pain and anxiety. Pneumonia and

atelectasis evolve more gradually, while heart failure shows fluid overload signs like crackles and edema, which are absent here.
SubChapter: Cardiopulmonary & Thromboembolic Complications

Q562. Answer: C

Explanation: Late postpartum bleeding with a firm uterus indicates retained placental tissue preventing vessel closure. Uterine atony causes a soft uterus, hematoma presents with localized pain and swelling, and DIC causes diffuse oozing unrelated to uterine tone. Surgical removal and antibiotics are required.
SubChapter: Hematologic & Hemorrhagic Disorders

Q563. Answer: A

Explanation: These classic signs indicate endometritis, an infection of the uterine lining after delivery. Immediate antibiotic therapy and provider notification are necessary to prevent septicemia. Ambulation, fluids, or ice offer limited benefit and delay essential treatment.
SubChapter: Infectious Conditions

Q564. Answer: A

Explanation: Severe hypertension and neurologic symptoms indicate postpartum preeclampsia, which can progress to eclampsia. Magnesium sulfate prevents seizures by stabilizing the nervous system. Methylergonovine raises blood pressure, worsening symptoms. Oxytocin and diuretics address other postpartum concerns but not seizure prevention.
SubChapter: Cardiopulmonary & Thromboembolic Complications

Q565. Answer: A

Explanation: Depressive symptoms lasting longer than two weeks meet criteria for postpartum depression and require professional evaluation. Delay in treatment risks worsening mental health and bonding impairment. Supportive measures alone are insufficient without therapy or medical management.
SubChapter: Psychological & Neurologic Conditions

Q566. Answer: D

Explanation: Disseminated intravascular coagulation results from clotting factor consumption following major hemorrhage or placental complications. It causes bleeding at multiple sites and abnormal coagulation studies. Anemia presents with pallor, not oozing; infection causes fever; thrombophlebitis leads to localized swelling.
SubChapter: Hematologic & Hemorrhagic Disorders

Q567. Answer: A

Explanation: Mastitis improves with frequent milk drainage and warm compresses, which promote circulation and healing. Stopping breastfeeding increases milk stasis and risk of abscess. Antibiotics compatible with breastfeeding are prescribed to treat Staphylococcus aureus infection.
SubChapter: Infectious Conditions

Q568. Answer: A

Explanation: Manic symptoms such as hyperactivity, decreased sleep, and impulsivity indicate postpartum psychosis with bipolar features. Depression presents with sadness; blues resolve quickly; anxiety lacks elevated mood or pressured speech. Immediate psychiatric evaluation is required for safety.
SubChapter: Psychological & Neurologic Conditions

Q569. Answer: A

Explanation: Hypothyroid phase of postpartum thyroiditis is characterized by high TSH and low T_4 levels. It follows the hyperthyroid phase and may persist for months. Other listed findings do not match endocrine patterns of postpartum thyroid dysfunction.
SubChapter: Metabolic & Endocrine Disorders

Q570. Answer: C

Explanation: Postpartum psychosis is a life-threatening emergency requiring immediate action to ensure safety and initiate psychiatric care. Reassurance or education alone risks maternal and infant harm. Urgent hospitalization and medication stabilization are essential.
SubChapter: Psychological & Neurologic Conditions

Q571. Answer: C

Explanation: Respiratory distress syndrome results from surfactant deficiency causing alveolar collapse, decreased lung compliance, and characteristic "ground-glass" radiograph. Option A—meconium aspiration occurs in term/post-term infants. Option B—transient tachypnea improves within 24 hours. Option D—PPHN features severe hypoxemia without diffuse opacity.
SubChapter: Cardiorespiratory Complications

Q572. Answer: A

Explanation: Choanal atresia blocks nasal airflow; neonates are obligate nasal breathers, so cyanosis worsens with feeding and improves when crying. Option B—coarctation causes poor femoral pulses, not nasal obstruction. Option C—tetralogy causes cyanosis during exertion. Option D—pulmonary hypoplasia presents with immediate distress unrelieved by crying.
SubChapter: Cardiorespiratory Complications

Q573. Answer: A

Explanation: Duodenal atresia results from failure of recanalization, commonly associated with trisomy 21, producing the classic "double-bubble" sign. Option B—pyloric stenosis develops weeks later. Option C—Hirschsprung causes distal obstruction with no meconium passage. Option D—meconium ileus occurs with cystic fibrosis, not Down syndrome.
SubChapter: Gastrointestinal Complications

Q574. Answer: B

Explanation: Rh incompatibility leads to maternal antibody-mediated hemolysis and anemia in affected neonates. Option C—ABO incompatibility is milder and often DAT-negative. Option A—G6PD deficiency produces episodic hemolysis after stress. Option D—physiologic jaundice appears later and lacks anemia.
SubChapter: Hematologic Complications

Q575. Answer: C

Explanation: Necrotizing enterocolitis requires immediate bowel rest, gastric decompression, and antibiotics to prevent perforation and sepsis. Option A—feeds worsen necrosis. Option B—is reserved for perforation or necrosis. Option D—acid suppression is not protective and may increase infection risk.
SubChapter: Gastrointestinal Complications

Q576. Answer: B

Explanation: Symptomatic hypoglycemia requires prompt IV dextrose to prevent neurologic injury. Option C—feeding is for mild, asymptomatic cases. Option A—oral sucrose treats procedural pain. Option D—glucagon is backup when IV access unavailable.
SubChapter: Endocrine Complications

Q577. Answer: B

Explanation: Early-onset neonatal sepsis requires immediate cultures and empiric IV ampicillin + gentamicin. Delay increases mortality. Option A—observation risks progression. Option C—antipyretics mask infection. Option D—waiting for fever is unsafe since neonates may be hypothermic.
SubChapter: Infectious Disease Complications

Q578. Answer: B

Explanation: Prostaglandin E1 maintains ductus arteriosus patency, allowing mixing between circuits in TGA. Option A—diuretics worsen hypotension. Option C—vasoconstriction reduces systemic flow. Option D—beta-blockers reduce contractility.
SubChapter: Cardiorespiratory Complications

Q579. Answer: B

Explanation: Caffeine citrate stimulates the central respiratory drive and decreases apnea frequency in preterm infants. Option A—depresses respiration. Option C—sedative that worsens apnea. Option D—anticonvulsant used for seizures, not apnea.
SubChapter: Neurologic Complications

Q580. Answer: A

Explanation: Severe coarctation may present after ductal closure with shock and acidosis; prostaglandin infusion restores systemic flow. Option B—VSD causes chronic heart failure, not acute collapse. Option C—ASD produces mild shunt. Option D—pulmonary stenosis primarily affects right-sided output.
SubChapter: Cardiorespiratory Complications

Q581. Answer: A

Explanation: Unconjugated hyperbilirubinemia may cross the blood-brain barrier, causing kernicterus with irreversible neurologic injury. Option B—anemia can accompany hemolysis but isn't the main threat. Option C—sepsis is separate etiology. Option D—dehydration worsens jaundice but isn't the cause of encephalopathy.
SubChapter: Hematologic Complications

Q582. Answer: B

Explanation: Prolonged membrane rupture increases risk of ascending infection and early-onset neonatal sepsis. Option A—reduces lung development, not infection risk. Option C—causes bleeding. Option D—causes fetal growth restriction, not bacterial exposure.
SubChapter: Infectious Disease Complications

Q583. Answer: B

Explanation: Neonatal abstinence syndrome results from in-utero opioid exposure leading to CNS irritability, GI upset, and autonomic dysfunction. Option A—causes jitteriness without GI symptoms. Option C—includes fever and hypotonia. Option D—presents with seizures, not rhythmic tremors and diarrhea.
SubChapter: Neurologic Complications

Q584. Answer: A

Explanation: A VSD produces a harsh holosystolic murmur and heart failure signs due to left-to-right shunt. Option B—murmur is continuous. Option C—systolic ejection murmur radiates to neck. Option D—causes weak femoral pulses, not holosystolic murmur.
SubChapter: Cardiorespiratory Complications

Q585. Answer: B

Explanation: Infants of diabetic mothers may have delayed surfactant production despite term gestation, causing respiratory distress syndrome. Option A—requires meconium staining. Option C—results from oligohydramnios or diaphragmatic hernia. Option D—resolves within 24 hours without severe hypoxemia.
SubChapter: Cardiorespiratory Complications

Q586. Answer: B

Explanation: Hirschsprung disease results from absence of enteric ganglion cells leading to functional obstruction and explosive stool after exam. Option A—temporary mucus plug clears easily. Option C—meconium ileus presents with thick meconium and no explosive release. Option D—causes narrow opening visible externally.
SubChapter: Gastrointestinal Complications

Q587. Answer: B

Explanation: Congenital rubella causes sensorineural deafness, cataracts, and patent ductus arteriosus ("classic triad"). Option A—causes chorioretinitis. Option C—produces periventricular calcifications. Option D—leads to snuffles and rash on palms/soles.
SubChapter: Infectious Disease Complications

Q588. Answer: C
Explanation: Infants of diabetic mothers often have transient hypocalcemia from suppressed parathyroid hormone synthesis due to maternal hypercalcemia. Option A—causes focal neurologic signs. Option B—would elevate infant calcium. Option D—may cause seizures but not selective hypocalcemia.
SubChapter: Endocrine Complications
Q589. Answer: B
Explanation: Anemia of prematurity results from inadequate erythropoietin response and short RBC lifespan. Option A—would increase reticulocytes. Option C—affects clotting, not RBCs. Option D—occurs after transfusions, not spontaneously.
SubChapter: Hematologic Complications
Q590. Answer: A
Explanation: 21-hydroxylase deficiency causes cortisol and aldosterone deficiency, salt-wasting crisis, and virilization. Option B—shows normal male hormones but female phenotype. Option C—presents with streak ovaries and normal electrolytes. Option D—has XXY karyotype with normal genitalia at birth.
SubChapter: Endocrine Complications
Q591. Answer: B
Explanation: CPAP maintains alveolar expansion in premature infants with surfactant deficiency, improving oxygenation and reducing mechanical-ventilation need. Option A—nitric oxide treats pulmonary hypertension. Option C—diuretics are for fluid overload. Option D—antibiotics address infection, not primary surfactant loss.
SubChapter: Cardiorespiratory Complications
Q592. Answer: A
Explanation: Esophageal atresia with TE fistula causes regurgitation and cyanosis when feeds enter the trachea; crying opens airway and improves color. Option B—vascular obstruction, not aspiration. Option C—chronic lung injury, not immediate distress. Option D—localized mass lesion.
SubChapter: Gastrointestinal Complications
Q593. Answer: B
Explanation: Anemia of prematurity arises from low erythropoietin and short RBC lifespan, producing mild anemia without hemolysis. Option A—occurs later and milder. Option C—produces positive Kleihauer-Betke test. Option D—shows episodic hemolysis after oxidative stress.
SubChapter: Hematologic Complications
Q594. Answer: C
Explanation: Group B Streptococcus is the leading cause of neonatal meningitis, producing hypoglycorrhachia and high protein. Option B—also causes sepsis but less common for meningitis. Option A—seen with maternal listeriosis. Option D—causes aseptic meningitis with normal glucose.
SubChapter: Infectious Complications
Q595. Answer: B
Explanation: Klinefelter syndrome (47,XXY) causes primary testicular failure leading to elevated gonadotropins and low testosterone. Option A—pituitary insufficiency. Option C—selective defects rare. Option D—not typical pattern.
SubChapter: Genetic/Endocrine Complications
Q596. Answer: B
Explanation: Pneumothorax causes air in pleural space, transilluminating brightly and leading to sudden desaturation. Option A—dense opacity on x-ray. Option C—collapsing segments without transillumination. Option D—fluid gives dull sound and no light transmission.
SubChapter: Cardiorespiratory Complications
Q597. Answer: B

Explanation: Bilious vomiting and gasless abdomen suggest midgut volvulus — a surgical emergency to prevent ischemia. Option A—contraindicated. Option C—delays treatment. Option D—dangerous as bowel necrosis progresses rapidly.
SubChapter: Gastrointestinal Complications

Q598. Answer: B

Explanation: Maternal IgG antibodies cross placenta and destroy fetal platelets in neonatal alloimmune thrombocytopenia or maternal ITP. Option A—marrow failure unlikely. Option C—produces lifelong defects. Option D—may contribute but not primary cause here.
SubChapter: Hematologic Complications

Q599. Answer: D

Explanation: Gonococcal ophthalmia appears within 48 hours after birth with profuse purulent discharge and eyelid edema, requiring urgent systemic therapy. Option A—presents later (5–14 days). Option C—milder. Option B—rare hospital-acquired infection.
SubChapter: Infectious Complications

Q600. Answer: B

Explanation: 21-hydroxylase deficiency impairs aldosterone synthesis, causing salt-wasting with hyponatremia and hyperkalemia. Option A—seen in Conn syndrome. Option C—unrelated. Option D—would exclude adrenal insufficiency.
SubChapter: Genetic/Endocrine Complications

Questions (601-700)

Q601. An infant receiving oxygen therapy for prematurity shows retinal vascular proliferation on exam. What is this condition?

A. Retinopathy of prematurity

B. Congenital glaucoma

C. Optic neuritis

D. Retinal hemorrhage

Q602. A newborn has dusky skin color and O_2 saturation 85% despite oxygen therapy. Hyperoxia test shows minimal PaO_2 change. What should be suspected?

A. Respiratory distress syndrome

B. Persistent pulmonary hypertension of the newborn

C. Transient tachypnea of the newborn

D. Pneumonia

Q603. A term infant develops projectile non-bilious vomiting at 3 weeks of age and palpable olive-shaped mass in epigastrium. Best treatment?

A. Metoclopramide therapy

B. Ramstedt pyloromyotomy

C. NPO and observe

D. Nasogastric lavage

Q604. A neonate develops severe pallor and tachycardia after delayed cord clamping. Placenta shows fetomaternal transfusion. What is most appropriate management?

A. Phototherapy

B. Packed RBC transfusion

C. Exchange transfusion

D. Iron supplement only

Q605. A 5-day-old infant presents with diffuse vesiculopustular rash and seizures. Maternal history: genital lesions late pregnancy. Most likely pathogen?

A. Varicella-zoster virus

B. Herpes simplex virus type 2

C. Cytomegalovirus

D. Human papillomavirus

Q606. A term infant has macroglossia, umbilical hernia, and hypoglycemia. Which syndrome is likely?

A. Prader-Willi syndrome

B. Edwards syndrome

C. Turner syndrome

D. Beckwith-Wiedemann syndrome

Q607. A preterm infant develops bradycardia and pallor with feedings. Cranial ultrasound reveals intraventricular hemorrhage. Which factor predisposed this infant?

A. Large for gestational age

B. Fragile germinal matrix vasculature

C. Polycythemia vera

D. Vitamin K deficiency

Q608. A 1-week-old infant shows progressive cyanosis and single loud S2. Prostaglandin E1 was started at birth. Which diagnosis is most likely?

A. Transposition of great arteries

B. Pulmonary atresia

C. Truncus arteriosus

D. Total anomalous pulmonary venous return

Q609. A neonate has bloody stools, distended abdomen, and pneumatosis intestinalis on x-ray. What is the most important initial management step?

A. Begin enteral feeds
B. Broad-spectrum antibiotics and bowel rest
C. Antacid therapy
D. Immediate surgery

Q610. A newborn male has ambiguous genitalia, hypertension, and low renin levels. Which enzyme deficiency causes this presentation?

A. 21-hydroxylase
B. 11β-hydroxylase
C. 17α-hydroxylase
D. 3β-hydroxysteroid dehydrogenase

Q611. A preterm infant presents with increased work of breathing, cyanosis, and decreased breath sounds on the right. Transillumination shows a bright glow. What is the likely diagnosis?

A. Pneumothorax
B. Pneumonia
C. Atelectasis
D. Pleural effusion

Q612. A newborn develops bilious vomiting within hours of birth. Abdominal x-ray shows a "double-bubble" sign with no gas distally. What condition is most likely?

A. Duodenal atresia
B. Pyloric stenosis
C. Malrotation without volvulus
D. Hirschsprung disease

Q613. A 33-week infant develops jaundice, hematocrit 22%, and elevated reticulocytes but a negative Coombs test. What is the likely cause?

A. Anemia of prematurity
B. ABO incompatibility
C. Rh hemolytic disease
D. Fetomaternal hemorrhage

Q614. A 2-day-old infant has lethargy, temperature instability, and poor feeding. Blood culture later grows Group B Streptococcus. What is the best empiric therapy before results?

A. Cefazolin alone
B. Vancomycin alone
C. Ampicillin and gentamicin
D. Ceftriaxone and azithromycin

Q615. A newborn girl presents with hypotonia, poor feeding, and low serum sodium and cortisol. ACTH levels are high. What disorder explains these findings?

A. Primary adrenal insufficiency
B. Pituitary hypoplasia
C. Congenital hypothyroidism
D. Adrenal hemorrhage

Q616. A preterm infant receiving mechanical ventilation shows chronic oxygen dependence and chest x-ray with alternating areas of lucency and fibrosis. What diagnosis fits best?

A. Bronchopulmonary dysplasia
B. Meconium aspiration syndrome
C. Persistent pulmonary hypertension

D. Pulmonary hypoplasia

Q617. A term infant develops abdominal distention and failure to pass meconium for > 48 hours. Rectal exam triggers explosive stool passage. What condition is suspected?

A. Hirschsprung disease

B. Meconium plug syndrome

C. Cystic fibrosis

D. Small-left-colon syndrome

Q618. A neonate with maternal history of untreated chorioamnionitis develops seizures and bulging fontanelle. Cerebrospinal fluid shows high protein and low glucose. What organism is most probable?

A. Enterovirus

B. Listeria monocytogenes

C. Escherichia coli

D. Group B Streptococcus

Q619. A 2-day-old infant has hypoglycemia, lethargy, and macroglossia. Physical exam reveals umbilical hernia. Which syndrome is consistent?

A. Beckwith-Wiedemann syndrome

B. Prader–Willi syndrome

C. Turner syndrome

D. Down syndrome

Q620. A ventilated preterm infant suddenly deteriorates with asymmetric chest expansion and hypotension. Needle decompression releases air hiss. Which pathophysiology occurred?

A. Tension pneumothorax

B. Pulmonary edema

C. Atelectasis

D. Pneumomediastinum

Q621. A preterm infant with NEC develops sudden abdominal wall redness and free air under diaphragm on x-ray. What action is required?

A. Emergency surgical exploration

B. Continue medical therapy only

C. Resume small feeds after 12 hours

D. Administer acetaminophen

Q622. A neonate has pallor, hypotension, and positive Kleihauer-Betke test showing fetal cells in maternal blood. What treatment is indicated?

A. Observation

B. Phototherapy

C. Iron supplementation alone

D. Packed red-cell transfusion

Q623. A 1-week-old infant shows irritability, poor feeding, and vesicular skin lesions. CSF PCR detects HSV-2. What is the best therapy?

A. Intravenous acyclovir

B. Oral fluconazole

C. Ampicillin and gentamicin

D. Topical antiseptic only

Q624. A newborn boy presents with severe hypoglycemia, hyperpigmented skin, and low cortisol with high ACTH. What condition is present?

A. Congenital adrenal hypoplasia

B. Congenital hypothyroidism

C. Pituitary adenoma

D. Pseudohypoaldosteronism

Q625. A preterm infant exhibits apnea and bradycardia spells that improve with gentle stimulation. Which medication prevents recurrence?

A. Caffeine citrate

B. Diazepam

C. Phenobarbital

D. Morphine

Q626. A neonate presents with continuous murmur at left upper sternal border and bounding pulses. What is the most likely defect?

A. Atrial septal defect

B. Ventricular septal defect

C. Patent ductus arteriosus

D. Pulmonary stenosis

Q627. A full-term infant has microcephaly, hepatosplenomegaly, and periventricular calcifications on imaging. Which infection is responsible?

A. Cytomegalovirus

B. Toxoplasmosis

C. Rubella

D. Herpes simplex virus

Q628. A newborn girl has low muscle tone, poor feeding, and enlarged tongue. TSH is elevated and T4 is low. What is the diagnosis?

A. Congenital hypothyroidism

B. Prader–Willi syndrome

C. Down syndrome

D. Beckwith-Wiedemann syndrome

Q629. A premature infant suddenly shows bradycardia and pallor during feeding. Cranial ultrasound reveals intraventricular hemorrhage. Which factor predisposed to this event?

A. Fragile germinal matrix vasculature

B. Polycythemia

C. Vitamin K deficiency

D. Excess oxygen therapy

Q630. A newborn develops cyanosis that worsens with feeding and improves with crying. Nasal passages cannot be catheterized. What is the diagnosis?

A. Subglottic stenosis

B. Pierre Robin sequence

C. Laryngomalacia

D. Choanal atresia

Q631. A 29-week gestation infant on CPAP develops increasing oxygen requirement, apnea, and diffuse bilateral hazy infiltrates on chest x-ray. Which intervention is most likely to reduce progression of surfactant deficiency?

A. Early caffeine therapy

B. Administer exogenous surfactant

C. Start oral feeds with donor milk

D. Begin empirical antibiotics

Q632. A term newborn exhibits copious oral secretions and episodes of coughing and cyanosis when attempts at feeding are made. Passage of an orogastric tube meets resistance in the upper chest. Most likely diagnosis?

A. Esophageal atresia with tracheoesophageal fistula

B. Laryngomalacia
C. Gastroesophageal reflux
D. Pierre Robin sequence

Q633. A 34-week infant has hematocrit 18%, tachycardia, and poor perfusion shortly after birth. Maternal history is unremarkable. What immediate diagnostic test helps confirm massive fetomaternal hemorrhage?

A. Direct Coombs test
B. Kleihauer-Betke test
C. Newborn bilirubin level
D. Maternal blood culture

Q634. A 12-hour-old neonate is febrile and irritable. Mother had prolonged rupture of membranes. Which empiric regimen is most appropriate immediately while awaiting cultures?

A. Ampicillin plus gentamicin
B. Oral azithromycin alone
C. Vancomycin alone
D. Ceftriaxone alone

Q635. A neonate presents with poor feeding, hypotension, hyponatremia, and hyperkalemia within the first week. Newborn screening shows markedly elevated 17-hydroxyprogesterone. What management step is urgent?

A. Begin stress-dose corticosteroids and fluid resuscitation
B. Start thyroid hormone replacement
C. Begin broad-spectrum antibiotics only
D. Start IV calcium gluconate

Q636. A preterm infant receiving supplemental oxygen and mechanical ventilation develops nasal flaring, retractions, and progressive chest wall fibrosis over weeks. Which long-term disorder is this infant at greatest risk for?

A. Bronchopulmonary dysplasia
B. Persistent pulmonary hypertension of the newborn
C. Meconium aspiration syndrome
D. Pulmonary sequestration

Q637. A full-term newborn has failure to pass meconium in the first 48 hours, abdominal distention, and a transition zone seen on contrast enema. What is the definitive diagnostic test?

A. Rectal biopsy demonstrating absence of ganglion cells
B. Sweat chloride test
C. Serum trypsinogen level
D. Abdominal ultrasound

Q638. A 3-day-old neonate with fever and lethargy has cerebrospinal fluid showing neutrophilic pleocytosis, low glucose, and high protein. Empiric therapy was started promptly. Which organism most commonly causes this presentation in term infants?

A. Enterovirus
B. Listeria monocytogenes
C. E. coli K1
D. Group B Streptococcus

Q639. A neonate demonstrates micrognathia, glossoptosis, and airway obstruction with cyanosis that improves when prone. What additional feeding concern is most likely?

A. Difficulty establishing effective latch and poor weight gain
B. Risk of necrotizing enterocolitis from early feeding
C. Excessive weight gain from overfeeding

D. High risk of urinary tract infection

Q640. A 7-day-old infant develops jaundice with a total bilirubin of 22 mg/dL and lethargy. Which neurotoxic complication is the highest concern if hyperbilirubinemia is untreated?

A. Acute bilirubin encephalopathy progressing to kernicterus

B. Neonatal stroke

C. Hypoxic-ischemic encephalopathy

D. Intraventricular hemorrhage

Q641. A premature infant shows redness, abdominal wall erythema, and pneumatosis intestinalis on x-ray. Blood cultures are pending. What initial steps should be taken?

A. NPO status, gastric decompression, IV antibiotics, and supportive care

B. Start trophic enteral feeds immediately

C. Begin immediate surgical resection without delay

D. Give high-dose oral probiotics and observe

Q642. A 10-day-old neonate shows conjunctivitis with mucopurulent discharge and eyelid edema. Which organism typically causes ophthalmia neonatorum within 48 hours of life and mandates systemic therapy?

A. Herpes simplex virus

B. Chlamydia trachomatis

C. Staphylococcus aureus

D. Neisseria gonorrhoeae

Q643. A term infant born to an insulin-dependent mother becomes jittery and has a blood glucose of 28 mg/dL. After initial IV dextrose, feeding is established. What physiologic mechanism explains the initial hypoglycemia?

A. Fetal hyperinsulinemia due to maternal hyperglycemia

B. Immature hepatic gluconeogenesis pathways

C. Inadequate glycogen stores from prematurity

D. Congenital hyperinsulinism unrelated to maternal diabetes

Q644. A 2-week-old infant has poor feeding, vomiting, and projectile nonbilious emesis with visible peristalsis and palpable olive-shaped mass. What electrolyte abnormality is most characteristic before treatment?

A. Hypochloremic metabolic alkalosis

B. Metabolic acidosis with hyperkalemia

C. Hyponatremic hyperkalemic metabolic acidosis

D. Respiratory alkalosis

Q645. A neonate presents with petechiae and platelet count of 15,000/μL shortly after birth. Mother has history of immune thrombocytopenia. What is the safest immediate approach?

A. Platelet transfusion if bleeding or very low count; monitor otherwise

B. Administer high-dose vitamin K only

C. Immediate exchange transfusion

D. Begin oral iron supplementation

Q646. A newborn develops apnea spells and generalized hypotonia; EEG and MRI confirm diffuse hypoxic-ischemic injury. Which long-term complication is most likely?

A. Pyloric stenosis

B. Chronic lung disease of prematurity

C. Retinopathy of prematurity

D. Cerebral palsy with motor impairment

Q647. A neonate with ambiguous genitalia is hyponatremic and hyperkalemic; 17-hydroxyprogesterone is elevated. Which long-term monitoring is essential for surviving infants?

A. Regular assessment of electrolytes and adrenal function, and growth monitoring
B. Routine MRI of the brain monthly
C. Frequent pulmonary function tests starting in neonatal period
D. Serial echocardiograms every week indefinitely

Q648. A ventilated preterm infant develops sudden unilateral scrotal swelling and systemic instability. Ultrasound shows intraperitoneal free fluid and testicular fluid collection. What is the probable diagnosis?
A. Spontaneous intestinal perforation with peritoneal fluid tracking
B. Testicular torsion unrelated to bowel pathology
C. Hydrocele due to patent processus vaginalis only
D. Incarcerated inguinal hernia only

Q649. A newborn develops fever, lethargy, and vesicular lesions; PCR from skin and CSF is positive for HSV-2. What is the recommended duration of intravenous antiviral therapy for CNS or disseminated disease?
A. 21 days of high-dose intravenous acyclovir
B. 5 days of oral acyclovir only
C. Single-dose intravenous acyclovir then observe
D. 7 days of topical acyclovir

Q650. A neonate shows severe hypoglycemia, hypotonia, and macroglossia; abdominal ultrasound detects an organomegaly. Which malignancy risk is increased and requires surveillance in infancy?
A. Leukemia with no organ surveillance needed
B. Neuroblastoma predominantly in extremities only
C. Retinoblastoma requiring weekly eye exams only
D. Hepatoblastoma and Wilms tumor risk, with abdominal tumor surveillance

Q651. A 30-week premature infant on mechanical ventilation suddenly develops asymmetrical breath sounds and bradycardia. Transillumination reveals a bright right-sided glow. What is the most likely diagnosis?
A. Pneumothorax
B. Pneumonia
C. Atelectasis
D. Pulmonary edema

Q652. A term newborn develops green, bilious vomiting and abdominal distention soon after birth. Radiograph shows no gas distal to the stomach. What is the likely diagnosis?
A. Duodenal atresia
B. Hirschsprung disease
C. Pyloric stenosis
D. Meconium ileus

Q653. A 2-day-old infant shows anemia, jaundice, and a positive direct antiglobulin test. The mother is Rh-negative. Which pathophysiologic mechanism explains these findings?
A. Maternal antibody-mediated hemolysis
B. Decreased erythropoietin production
C. Fetal blood loss during delivery
D. Enzyme deficiency causing RBC fragility

Q654. A premature infant becomes lethargic, hypothermic, and develops respiratory distress. Blood culture reveals E. coli. Which maternal condition most increases this risk?
A. Maternal hypertension
B. Polyhydramnios
C. Placenta previa

D. Prolonged rupture of membranes

Q655. A newborn with ambiguous genitalia has hyponatremia and hyperkalemia. Serum 17-hydroxyprogesterone is markedly elevated. What is the best initial management?

A. Intravenous fluids with corticosteroid replacement
B. Immediate thyroid hormone therapy
C. Oral calcium supplementation
D. Observation without intervention

Q656. A preterm infant treated with high-concentration oxygen develops retinopathy of prematurity. Which preventive measure reduces this complication?

A. Careful titration to maintain target oxygen saturation range
B. Routine use of 100% oxygen in resuscitation
C. Vitamin A supplementation only
D. Complete avoidance of oxygen therapy

Q657. A 1-week-old infant has abdominal distention and bloody stools; x-ray reveals pneumatosis intestinalis. What immediate step should be taken?

A. Stop feeds, decompress stomach, start broad-spectrum antibiotics
B. Begin small oral feeds to stimulate bowel motility
C. Give proton-pump inhibitors
D. Observe for 24 hours without treatment

Q658. A neonate exposed to untreated maternal syphilis presents with nasal discharge, hepatosplenomegaly, and a maculopapular rash including palms and soles. What test confirms diagnosis?

A. Elevated liver enzymes only
B. Negative direct Coombs test
C. Normal cerebrospinal-fluid VDRL
D. Positive fluorescent treponemal antibody absorption (FTA-ABS) test

Q659. A term infant of a diabetic mother develops hypoglycemia and jitteriness within an hour after birth. What physiological process explains this finding?

A. Persistent fetal hyperinsulinemia after maternal glucose supply stops
B. Inadequate glycogen stores due to prematurity
C. Impaired gluconeogenesis from liver immaturity
D. Low cortisol levels after delivery

Q660. A ventilated neonate develops sudden hypotension and asymmetric chest movement. Needle aspiration produces air under pressure. What complication occurred?

A. Tension pneumothorax
B. Pneumomediastinum
C. Atelectasis
D. Pleural effusion

Q661. A newborn fails to pass meconium for 72 hours and has a distended abdomen. Contrast enema shows microcolon and thick inspissated stool. Which condition is likely?

A. Meconium ileus due to cystic fibrosis
B. Hirschsprung disease
C. Duodenal atresia
D. Small-left-colon syndrome

Q662. A 3-day-old neonate has a platelet count < 30 000/µL but no bleeding. Mother has idiopathic thrombocytopenic purpura. Appropriate management?

A. Give prophylactic antibiotics
B. Immediate exchange transfusion

C. Start high-dose iron supplementation
D. Monitor closely; transfuse platelets if bleeding or count < 20 000/μL

Q663. A 2-week-old infant presents with vesicular rash and seizures. HSV-2 infection is confirmed. Which treatment plan is recommended?
A. Intravenous acyclovir for 21 days with follow-up CSF PCR
B. Topical antiviral ointment only
C. Oral acyclovir for 5 days
D. Empiric broad-spectrum antibiotics

Q664. A newborn girl has large tongue, umbilical hernia, and macrosomia. Glucose readings remain low. Which long-term surveillance is essential?
A. Abdominal ultrasound for Wilms tumor and hepatoblastoma
B. Annual echocardiogram for congenital heart disease
C. Routine head MRI for structural anomalies
D. No follow-up once glucose normalizes

Q665. A preterm infant on high oxygen develops chronic lung changes. Which therapy helps prevent progression of bronchopulmonary dysplasia?
A. Minimizing oxygen concentration and gentle ventilation strategies
B. Continuous high PEEP levels
C. Routine corticosteroids from birth
D. Immediate cessation of all respiratory support

Q666. A term newborn presents with inspiratory stridor worsening when supine and improving when prone. Oxygen saturation is normal. What is the probable cause?
A. Laryngomalacia
B. Tracheoesophageal fistula
C. Vocal-cord paralysis
D. Choanal atresia

Q667. A 5-day-old infant becomes hypotonic with poor feeding and temperature instability. CSF shows elevated protein and low glucose. Which organism should be suspected?
A. Enterovirus
B. Listeria monocytogenes
C. Staphylococcus aureus
D. Candida albicans

Q668. A neonate has tremors, high-pitched cry, and sneezing within 48 hours of birth. The mother used opioids during pregnancy. What is the preferred management?
A. Supportive care with swaddling and small frequent feeds
B. Immediate anticonvulsant therapy
C. Restrict fluids and stimulate frequently
D. Withhold feeds until symptoms resolve

Q669. A 2-day-old infant has persistent cyanosis unresponsive to oxygen and a single loud S2. Echocardiogram confirms transposition of the great arteries. What treatment maintains systemic oxygenation before surgery?
A. Continuous prostaglandin E1 infusion
B. High-dose furosemide
C. Beta-blocker infusion
D. Diaphragmatic pacing

Q670. A preterm infant with periventricular leukomalacia is at increased risk for which developmental outcome?
A. Spastic cerebral palsy

B. Muscular dystrophy
C. Autism spectrum disorder
D. Congenital myasthenia

Q671. A newborn delivered by cesarean section exhibits tachypnea and mild retractions without cyanosis two hours after birth. Which condition is most likely?
A. Respiratory distress syndrome
B. Meconium aspiration syndrome
C. Transient tachypnea of the newborn (TTN)
D. Pneumothorax

Q672. A term infant presents with grunting, nasal flaring, and cyanosis immediately after birth. Chest X-ray shows ground-glass appearance. What is the most likely diagnosis?
A. Respiratory distress syndrome (RDS)
B. Transient tachypnea of the newborn
C. Persistent pulmonary hypertension
D. Pneumonia

Q673. A 38-week infant born through meconium-stained amniotic fluid has respiratory distress and coarse crackles. What is the priority nursing intervention?
A. Provide oxygen and prepare for mechanical ventilation
B. Stimulate the infant to cry
C. Delay suctioning until stable
D. Administer antibiotics immediately

Q674. A newborn becomes cyanotic when feeding but pink when crying. What congenital condition is suspected?
A. Choanal atresia
B. Cystic fibrosis
C. Laryngomalacia
D. Pneumothorax

Q675. A preterm infant at 32 weeks develops periodic apnea lasting 25 seconds with bradycardia and desaturation. What is the first nursing action?
A. Administer oxygen only
B. Begin chest compressions immediately
C. Gently stimulate the infant and assess respirations
D. Notify the provider before intervening

Q676. A neonate of a diabetic mother becomes jittery and lethargic two hours after birth. Blood glucose is 28 mg/dL. What should the nurse do first?
A. Feed the infant with breast milk or formula
B. Start IV dextrose infusion immediately
C. Recheck glucose in 30 minutes
D. Wrap the infant to maintain warmth only

Q677. A term newborn exhibits pallor, tachycardia, and hematocrit of 28%. Which cause should be suspected first first?
A. Fetomaternal hemorrhage
B. Polycythemia
C. Hypoglycemia
D. Hyperbilirubinemia

Q678. A 2-day-old infant has total bilirubin of 16 mg/dL and visible jaundice to the legs. What is the appropriate nursing action?
A. Initiate phototherapy

B. Observe and repeat bilirubin in 12 hours
C. Begin IV fluids only
D. Apply sunlight exposure near a window

Q679. A newborn exhibits poor feeding, temperature instability, and lethargy on day three. Which laboratory test should be prioritized?
A. Serum bilirubin
B. Complete blood count
C. Blood glucose
D. Blood culture

Q680. A neonate born to a mother with untreated chorioamnionitis presents with temperature instability and mottled skin. What is the priority nursing intervention?
A. Start IV antibiotics as prescribed after cultures
B. Observe closely and record temperature hourly
C. Delay antibiotics until WBC results return
D. Apply external warmth and monitor

Q681. A preterm infant displays continuous seizures, hypotonia, and poor feeding after a difficult delivery with hypoxia. What condition should the nurse suspect?
A. Hypoxic-ischemic encephalopathy
B. Neonatal hypoglycemia
C. Intraventricular hemorrhage
D. Metabolic alkalosis

Q682. A nurse notes a newborn's temperature is 35.5°C (95.9°F) and the infant is pale and lethargic. What is the first action?
A. Place the infant under a radiant warmer
B. Feed the infant immediately
C. Apply cold stress protocol with blankets
D. Assess for infection only

Q683. A term newborn develops tachypnea, cyanosis, and loud systolic murmur unresponsive to oxygen. Echocardiography shows right-to-left shunting. Which condition is indicated?
A. Patent ductus arteriosus
B. Transient tachypnea of the newborn
C. Ventricular septal defect
D. Persistent pulmonary hypertension of the newborn (PPHN)

Q684. A newborn has seizures, jaundice, and hepatosplenomegaly. The mother reports a history of cytomegalovirus infection. Which diagnosis is most consistent?
A. Congenital CMV infection
B. Neonatal hypoglycemia
C. Erythroblastosis fetalis
D. Toxoplasmosis

Q685. A 36-hour-old term infant shows irritability, poor feeding, and high-pitched cry after maternal narcotic use. What therapy is indicated?
A. Initiate neonatal abstinence management protocol
B. Provide extra stimulation to soothe
C. Restrict feedings to avoid vomiting
D. Observe only unless seizures occur

Q686. A newborn's hematocrit is 70%, and the infant appears plethoric with sluggish capillary refill. Which management step is indicated?
A. Partial exchange transfusion

B. Observation only
C. Increase iron supplementation
D. Phototherapy

Q687. A premature neonate has weak cry, hypotonia, and poor thermoregulation after birth. What is the nurse's immediate priority?
A. Stimulate to cry
B. Start IV glucose
C. Maintain neutral thermal environment
D. Administer antibiotics prophylactically

Q688. A newborn has a continuous harsh murmur and bounding pulses. What congenital condition is suspected?
A. Patent ductus arteriosus
B. Ventricular septal defect
C. Coarctation of the aorta
D. Tetralogy of Fallot

Q689. A newborn delivered after shoulder dystocia has absent movement in the right arm but good hand grasp. Which nerve injury is indicated?
A. Erb's palsy
B. Klumpke's palsy
C. Phrenic nerve injury
D. Facial nerve palsy

Q690. A neonate becomes lethargic with respiratory distress, poor feeding, and hypothermia at 24 hours old. Maternal history includes group B streptococcal colonization. What is the likely diagnosis?
A. Early-onset neonatal sepsis
B. Late-onset sepsis
C. TTN
D. Hypoglycemia only

Q691. A preterm neonate at 30 weeks develops progressive apnea, bradycardia, and pallor. Which intervention should be implemented first?
A. Notify physician before action
B. Start chest compressions immediately
C. Administer IV caffeine
D. Gentle tactile stimulation and airway assessment

Q692. A 34-week infant on oxygen therapy suddenly develops asymmetrical chest expansion, diminished breath sounds on the right, and desaturation. What should the nurse suspect?
A. Pneumothorax
B. Bronchopulmonary dysplasia
C. Respiratory distress syndrome
D. Atelectasis

Q693. A term newborn shows generalized cyanosis unresponsive to oxygen, loud systolic murmur, and boot-shaped heart on X-ray. Which congenital condition is likely?
A. Tetralogy of Fallot
B. Ventricular septal defect
C. Patent ductus arteriosus
D. Coarctation of the aorta

Q694. A newborn exhibits lethargy, poor feeding, and tremors. Blood glucose is 22 mg/dL. What is the immediate nursing action?
A. Begin IV dextrose infusion

B. Encourage breastfeeding
C. Monitor glucose hourly only
D. Provide warm environment

Q695. A 36-hour-old newborn with Rh incompatibility presents with rising bilirubin levels and anemia. What treatment should the nurse anticipate?
A. IV fluids only
B. Phototherapy alone
C. Exchange transfusion
D. Iron supplementation

Q696. A neonate exposed to maternal Group B Streptococcus develops respiratory distress, temperature instability, and hypotension within 12 hours of birth. What should the nurse do first?
A. Obtain cultures and start IV antibiotics
B. Observe for 24 hours before starting antibiotics
C. Delay antibiotics until CBC results return
D. Place infant under warmer and monitor

Q697. A term infant is noted to have jitteriness, high-pitched cry, and frequent yawning. The mother reports opioid use during pregnancy. What is the likely diagnosis?
A. Neonatal abstinence syndrome
B. Hypoglycemia
C. Sepsis
D. Cerebral palsy

Q698. A newborn has persistent jaundice at two weeks of age, clay-colored stools, and dark urine. Which condition should the nurse suspect?
A. Biliary atresia
B. Physiologic jaundice
C. Breast milk jaundice
D. Hemolytic anemia

Q699. A newborn presents with temperature 34.8°C (94.6°F), weak cry, and respiratory distress. Which complication is most likely developing?
A. Respiratory alkalosis
B. Sepsis from hypothermia
C. Hypoglycemia only
D. Cold stress leading to metabolic acidosis

Q700. A neonate with Down syndrome has poor feeding, tachypnea, and hepatomegaly. Echocardiography reveals complete atrioventricular canal defect. What is the primary nursing focus?
A. Support adequate nutrition and prevent heart failure
B. Encourage vigorous feeding to gain weight
C. Restrict fluids completely
D. Delay medical follow-up until six months

Answer key and Explanation (601-700)

Q601. Answer: A

Explanation: Retinopathy of prematurity results from oxygen-induced vasoconstriction followed by abnormal neovascularization after hypoxia. Option B—causes enlarged cornea. Option C—rare in neonates. Option D—traumatic finding at delivery.

SubChapter: Neurologic Complications

Q602. Answer: B

Explanation: Persistent pulmonary hypertension causes right-to-left shunting with minimal oxygen response on hyperoxia test. Option A—improves with oxygen. Option C—resolves quickly. Option D—shows infectious symptoms and infiltrates.

SubChapter: Cardiorespiratory Complications

Q603. Answer: B

Explanation: Hypertrophic pyloric stenosis requires surgical pyloromyotomy after electrolyte correction. Option A—ineffective. Option C—does not resolve obstruction. Option D—temporary relief only.

SubChapter: Gastrointestinal Complications

Q604. Answer: B

Explanation: Acute fetomaternal hemorrhage causes severe anemia requiring packed RBC transfusion to restore oxygen carrying capacity. Option A—treats jaundice only. Option C—for hyperbilirubinemia, not volume loss. Option D—insufficient for acute loss.

SubChapter: Hematologic Complications

Q605. Answer: B

Explanation: Neonatal HSV-2 infection presents with vesicular lesions, sepsis-like illness, and CNS involvement. Prompt acyclovir therapy reduces mortality. Option A—produces congenital scarring. Option C—causes sensorineural loss and calcifications. Option D—non-ulcerative warts.

SubChapter: Infectious Complications

Q606. Answer: D

Explanation: Beckwith-Wiedemann syndrome involves overgrowth, macroglossia, organomegaly, and neonatal hypoglycemia due to hyperinsulinism. Option A—hypotonia and poor growth. Option C—webbed neck and short stature. Option B—trisomy 18 with micrognathia and clenched hands.

SubChapter: Genetic/Endocrine Complications

Q607. Answer: B

Explanation: Premature infants have fragile germinal matrix vessels that rupture from fluctuating cerebral blood flow. Option A—unrelated. Option C—rare in newborns. Option D—causes bleeding elsewhere but not typical site.

SubChapter: Neurologic Complications

Q608. Answer: A

Explanation: Transposition of great arteries causes parallel circulations and ductal dependence; prostaglandin keeps ductus open for mixing until surgery. Option B—no main pulmonary outflow. Option C—single trunk with murmur. Option D—pulmonary veins to RA with different findings.

SubChapter: Cardiorespiratory Complications

Q609. Answer: B

Explanation: Necrotizing enterocolitis requires cessation of feeds, gastric decompression, and IV antibiotics. Option A—aggravates disease. Option C—not effective. Option D—for perforation or failure of medical management.

SubChapter: Gastrointestinal Complications

Q610. Answer: B

Explanation: 11β-hydroxylase deficiency increases deoxycorticosterone (a mineralocorticoid), causing hypertension and virilization. Option A—causes salt-wasting and hypotension. Option C—produces hypertension with underdeveloped genitalia. Option D—rare, affects early steroid synthesis.
SubChapter: Genetic/Endocrine Complications

Q611. Answer: A

Explanation: Air leaking into the pleural space produces a pneumothorax, seen as a bright glow on transillumination and diminished breath sounds. Pneumonia would cause crackles and infiltrates. Atelectasis shows reduced volume without transillumination. Pleural effusion creates dullness and poor light transmission.
SubChapter: Cardiorespiratory Complications

Q612. Answer: A

Explanation: Duodenal atresia causes proximal obstruction from failure of recanalization, producing the characteristic double-bubble appearance. Pyloric stenosis occurs later with non-bilious emesis. Malrotation usually has variable gas distribution. Hirschsprung disease manifests with delayed meconium passage rather than immediate bilious vomiting.
SubChapter: Gastrointestinal Complications

Q613. Answer: A

Explanation: Anemia of prematurity results from inadequate erythropoietin response and shortened red-cell lifespan. ABO and Rh incompatibilities cause positive Coombs tests. Fetomaternal hemorrhage produces acute anemia with signs of blood loss rather than gradual decline.
SubChapter: Hematologic Complications

Q614. Answer: C

Explanation: Ampicillin with gentamicin provides broad coverage for Group B Streptococcus and Gram-negative organisms in early-onset neonatal sepsis. Vancomycin or cefazolin alone would miss Gram-negative pathogens. Ceftriaxone can displace bilirubin, risking kernicterus in neonates.
SubChapter: Infectious Complications

Q615. Answer: A

Explanation: Primary adrenal insufficiency causes cortisol and aldosterone deficiency with high ACTH. Pituitary hypoplasia would show low ACTH. Congenital hypothyroidism mainly causes macroglossia and lethargy. Adrenal hemorrhage presents with abdominal mass and anemia rather than persistent electrolyte imbalance.
SubChapter: Genetic/Endocrine Complications

Q616. Answer: A

Explanation: Bronchopulmonary dysplasia is chronic lung injury from prolonged ventilation and oxygen exposure, producing patchy atelectasis and fibrosis. Meconium aspiration occurs in term infants. Pulmonary hypertension shows right-to-left shunting. Pulmonary hypoplasia results from structural underdevelopment, not fibrosis.
SubChapter: Cardiorespiratory Complications

Q617. Answer: A

Explanation: Hirschsprung disease arises from absence of enteric ganglion cells, causing functional obstruction relieved transiently after rectal exam. Meconium plug and small-left-colon syndromes are transient. Cystic fibrosis produces thick meconium ileus, not explosive release.
SubChapter: Gastrointestinal Complications

Q618. Answer: D

Explanation: Group B Streptococcus is the commonest cause of early-onset neonatal meningitis, especially following maternal chorioamnionitis. Listeria and E. coli may cause similar signs but are less frequent. Enteroviral infection usually has normal glucose and milder symptoms.
SubChapter: Infectious Complications

Q619. Answer: A
Explanation: Beckwith-Wiedemann syndrome features macrosomia, macroglossia, organomegaly, and neonatal hypoglycemia from hyperinsulinism. Prader–Willi syndrome causes hypotonia and feeding difficulty. Turner syndrome presents in females with short stature. Down syndrome is associated with hypotonia and duodenal atresia but not hypoglycemia.
SubChapter: Genetic/Endocrine Complications
Q620. Answer: A
Explanation: A tension pneumothorax traps air under pressure, shifting mediastinum and impairing venous return; decompression rapidly relieves distress. Pulmonary edema shows crackles and frothy sputum. Atelectasis causes gradual desaturation. Pneumomediastinum gives subcutaneous crepitus, not hemodynamic collapse.
SubChapter: Cardiorespiratory Complications
Q621. Answer: A
Explanation: Perforation from necrotizing enterocolitis demands immediate surgical intervention to prevent sepsis and death. Medical therapy alone is inadequate once pneumoperitoneum appears. Resuming feeds or using analgesics without surgery risks fatal peritonitis.
SubChapter: Gastrointestinal Complications
Q622. Answer: D
Explanation: Acute fetomaternal hemorrhage causes severe anemia requiring immediate packed RBC transfusion to restore oxygen delivery. Phototherapy treats hyperbilirubinemia, not volume loss. Iron supplementation corrects stores long-term but not acute shock. Observation alone endangers survival.
SubChapter: Hematologic Complications
Q623. Answer: A
Explanation: Neonatal herpes requires high-dose intravenous acyclovir to prevent CNS damage and death. Antifungals or antibiotics do not target HSV. Topical agents cannot control systemic infection.
SubChapter: Infectious Complications
Q624. Answer: A
Explanation: Congenital adrenal hypoplasia leads to primary adrenal failure, causing cortisol deficiency, hypoglycemia, and skin hyperpigmentation from high ACTH. Hypothyroidism causes macroglossia but normal ACTH. Pituitary adenoma is rare in newborns. Pseudohypoaldosteronism presents with salt wasting but normal cortisol.
SubChapter: Genetic/Endocrine Complications
Q625. Answer: A
Explanation: Caffeine citrate stimulates respiratory drive and reduces apneic episodes in premature infants. Sedatives such as diazepam, phenobarbital, or morphine depress respiration and can exacerbate apnea.
SubChapter: Neurologic Complications
Q626. Answer: C
Explanation: Patent ductus arteriosus produces a continuous machinery murmur and bounding pulses from left-to-right shunt. A ventricular septal defect is holosystolic, atrial septal defect is soft and fixed-split S2, and pulmonary stenosis gives a systolic ejection murmur.
SubChapter: Cardiorespiratory Complications
Q627. Answer: A
Explanation: Congenital cytomegalovirus infection causes microcephaly, jaundice, and periventricular calcifications. Toxoplasmosis produces diffuse calcifications and chorioretinitis. Rubella leads to cataracts and PDA. Herpes simplex causes vesicular rash and meningoencephalitis.
SubChapter: Infectious Complications
Q628. Answer: A

Explanation: Congenital hypothyroidism presents with hypotonia, macroglossia, and prolonged jaundice; screening shows high TSH and low T4. Prader–Willi syndrome has normal thyroid levels. Down syndrome causes similar features but normal hormones. Beckwith-Wiedemann is an overgrowth syndrome.
SubChapter: Genetic/Endocrine Complications

Q629. Answer: A

Explanation: Preterm infants have fragile germinal matrix capillaries susceptible to rupture from hemodynamic fluctuations. Polycythemia thickens blood but rarely causes bleeding. Vitamin K deficiency affects coagulation systemically. Oxygen therapy contributes to ROP not IVH.
SubChapter: Neurologic Complications

Q630. Answer: D

Explanation: Choanal atresia causes obstruction of posterior nares; because newborns are obligate nasal breathers, cyanosis worsens during feeding and improves with crying. Pierre Robin sequence presents with micrognathia and glossoptosis. Laryngomalacia and subglottic stenosis produce stridor but allow nasal airflow.
SubChapter: Cardiorespiratory Complications

Q631. Answer: B

Explanation: Administering exogenous surfactant directly addresses surfactant deficiency in very preterm infants, improving lung compliance and oxygenation. Caffeine helps apnea but not surfactant production. Oral feeds do not treat respiratory insufficiency, and antibiotics are for suspected infection rather than primary surfactant deficiency.
SubChapter: Cardiorespiratory Complications

Q632. Answer: A

Explanation: Esophageal atresia with tracheoesophageal fistula presents with drooling, choking with feeds, and inability to pass a tube into the stomach; aspiration risk is high. Laryngomalacia causes inspiratory stridor but tube passage is normal. Reflux does not obstruct tube passage. Pierre Robin includes micrognathia and airway obstruction.
SubChapter: Gastrointestinal Complications

Q633. Answer: B

Explanation: The Kleihauer-Betke test detects fetal red blood cells in maternal circulation and is useful to confirm fetomaternal hemorrhage causing acute neonatal anemia. A direct Coombs test identifies immune hemolysis. Bilirubin level and maternal blood cultures are informative for other issues but not diagnostic for fetomaternal hemorrhage.
SubChapter: Hematologic Complications

Q634. Answer: A

Explanation: Ampicillin plus gentamicin provides broad empiric coverage for common early-onset pathogens including Group B Streptococcus and Gram-negative bacilli in neonates with risk factors like prolonged rupture of membranes. Monotherapy with vancomycin or third-generation cephalosporins is suboptimal as initial empiric therapy for early neonatal sepsis.
SubChapter: Infectious Complications

Q635. Answer: A

Explanation: Elevated 17-hydroxyprogesterone suggests congenital adrenal hyperplasia with salt-wasting; urgent fluid resuscitation and glucocorticoid (and mineralocorticoid) replacement stabilize electrolytes and blood pressure while endocrine evaluation proceeds. Thyroid replacement, antibiotics, or calcium address different emergencies and will not correct adrenal crisis.
SubChapter: Genetic/Endocrine Complications

Q636. Answer: A

Explanation: Prolonged oxygen therapy and mechanical ventilation in preterm infants injures developing lungs and predisposes to bronchopulmonary dysplasia, characterized by chronic oxygen dependence and

radiographic fibrosis. Persistent pulmonary hypertension is an acute transitional disorder. Meconium aspiration and sequestration are distinct etiologies unrelated to prolonged ventilator-induced injury.
SubChapter: Cardiorespiratory Complications

Q637. Answer: A

Explanation: A rectal biopsy showing absence of submucosal and myenteric ganglion cells confirms Hirschsprung disease and guides surgical planning. Sweat testing and trypsinogen are used in cystic fibrosis diagnosis. Ultrasound may assist but cannot demonstrate aganglionosis definitively.
SubChapter: Gastrointestinal Complications

Q638. Answer: D

Explanation: Group B Streptococcus remains the leading cause of early-onset bacterial meningitis in term neonates, producing neutrophilic CSF with low glucose and high protein; prompt empiric antibiotics are critical. Listeria and E. coli can also cause neonatal meningitis but are less frequent in term infants; enterovirus typically causes aseptic meningitis with normal glucose.
SubChapter: Infectious Complications

Q639. Answer: A

Explanation: Micrognathia and glossoptosis, characteristic of Pierre Robin sequence, impair oral feeding and swallowing, leading to poor latch and weight gain; feeding strategies and possible tube feeding are often required. NEC, overfeeding, and urinary infections are not specific feeding complications of this condition.
SubChapter: Neurologic/GI Complications

Q640. Answer: A

Explanation: Severe unconjugated hyperbilirubinemia can lead to acute bilirubin encephalopathy and permanent kernicterus with dystonia and hearing loss. Stroke, hypoxic-ischemic injury, and IVH are important neonatal neurologic problems but are not sequelae of untreated unconjugated hyperbilirubinemia.
SubChapter: Hematologic Complications

Q641. Answer: A

Explanation: Necrotizing enterocolitis management begins with bowel rest, decompression, broad-spectrum IV antibiotics, and supportive care while monitoring for perforation; surgery is reserved for perforation or clinical deterioration. Early enteral feeds, unproven probiotic monotherapy, or immediate resection without stabilization are inappropriate initial steps.
SubChapter: Gastrointestinal Complications

Q642. Answer: D

Explanation: Neisseria gonorrhoeae causes early-onset, fulminant neonatal conjunctivitis within 24–48 hours, often with copious purulent discharge and eyelid swelling; systemic antibiotic therapy is required to prevent complications. Chlamydial conjunctivitis typically presents later, and staphylococcal or viral causes have different courses and treatments.
SubChapter: Infectious Complications

Q643. Answer: A

Explanation: Maternal hyperglycemia stimulates fetal insulin production; after birth, loss of maternal glucose supply combined with persistent neonatal hyperinsulinemia causes hypoglycemia. Immature gluconeogenesis and prematurity also contribute, but fetal hyperinsulinemia from maternal diabetes is the primary mechanism in infants of diabetic mothers.
SubChapter: Endocrine Complications

Q644. Answer: A

Explanation: Pyloric stenosis leads to vomiting of gastric acid, causing loss of hydrogen and chloride and resulting in hypochloremic, hypokalemic metabolic alkalosis. This metabolic disturbance is classic and

must be corrected before surgical pyloromyotomy. Other listed disturbances do not match the pathophysiology.
SubChapter: Gastrointestinal Complications

Q645. Answer: A

Explanation: Neonatal thrombocytopenia due to maternal antibodies may be severe; platelet transfusion is indicated for significant bleeding or extremely low counts, while stable infants can be closely monitored. Vitamin K, exchange transfusion, or iron do not address immune-mediated platelet destruction acutely.
SubChapter: Hematologic Complications

Q646. Answer: D

Explanation: Moderate to severe hypoxic-ischemic encephalopathy often results in long-term neurodevelopmental impairment, including cerebral palsy, cognitive deficits, and seizure disorders. Chronic lung disease, ROP, and pyloric stenosis are unrelated sequelae of perinatal hypoxia in different contexts.
SubChapter: Neurologic Complications

Q647. Answer: A

Explanation: In congenital adrenal hyperplasia, ongoing monitoring of electrolytes, adrenal hormones, and growth is crucial to manage salt-wasting episodes and optimize hormone replacement; brain MRI, pulmonary tests, and serial cardiac imaging are not routinely required without specific indications.
SubChapter: Genetic/Endocrine Complications

Q648. Answer: A

Explanation: In extremely low birth weight infants, spontaneous intestinal perforation can produce free intraperitoneal fluid that tracks into the scrotum via a patent processus vaginalis, presenting with scrotal swelling and instability. Isolated testicular torsion, simple hydrocele, or a reducible hernia would not typically cause systemic instability and free intraperitoneal fluid.
SubChapter: Gastrointestinal Complications

Q649. Answer: A

Explanation: Neonatal HSV with central nervous system or disseminated involvement requires prolonged high-dose intravenous acyclovir, typically for 21 days, to reduce mortality and long-term neurologic impairment. Short courses, topical therapy, or single doses are inadequate for systemic neonatal HSV disease.
SubChapter: Infectious Complications

Q650. Answer: D

Explanation: Overgrowth syndromes such as Beckwith-Wiedemann increase the risk for embryonal tumors including hepatoblastoma and Wilms tumor; surveillance with periodic abdominal ultrasound and AFP measurements during infancy is recommended. Neuroblastoma, retinoblastoma, and leukemia have different screening protocols and risk profiles.
SubChapter: Genetic/Endocrine Complications

Q651. Answer: A

Explanation: Air leakage into the pleural space causes pneumothorax, presenting with decreased breath sounds, bradycardia, and a bright transillumination sign. Pneumonia produces crackles and fever. Atelectasis results in dullness, not transillumination. Pulmonary edema leads to diffuse rales and bilateral findings.
SubChapter: Cardiorespiratory Complications

Q652. Answer: A

Explanation: Duodenal atresia results from failure of recanalization, producing early bilious vomiting and the classic “double-bubble” appearance. Hirschsprung disease causes delayed meconium passage.

Pyloric stenosis is non-bilious and later onset. Meconium ileus occurs in cystic fibrosis and shows multiple air-fluid levels.
SubChapter: Gastrointestinal Complications

Q653. Answer: A

Explanation: Rh incompatibility allows maternal anti-D antibodies to destroy fetal red blood cells, producing hemolytic anemia and jaundice. Reduced erythropoietin or enzyme deficiency do not yield a positive Coombs test. Fetomaternal hemorrhage would show acute blood loss without immune evidence.
SubChapter: Hematologic Complications

Q654. Answer: D

Explanation: Early-onset neonatal sepsis with E. coli often follows prolonged rupture of membranes that allows ascending infection. Polyhydramnios is unrelated to infection. Placenta previa leads to bleeding, not sepsis. Hypertension causes growth restriction but not infection predisposition.
SubChapter: Infectious Complications

Q655. Answer: A

Explanation: The presentation indicates salt-wasting congenital adrenal hyperplasia; urgent isotonic fluids and hydrocortisone restore hemodynamic stability. Thyroid or calcium therapy does not correct adrenal crisis. Observation alone risks circulatory collapse.
SubChapter: Genetic/Endocrine Complications

Q656. Answer: A

Explanation: Maintaining oxygen saturation within recommended limits prevents hyperoxia-induced vasoconstriction that triggers retinopathy. Constant high oxygen exposure increases risk, whereas complete avoidance causes hypoxia. Vitamin A helps lung development but does not prevent retinal neovascularization.
SubChapter: Neurologic Complications

Q657. Answer: A

Explanation: Necrotizing enterocolitis demands bowel rest, decompression, IV antibiotics, and close monitoring. Continued feeds or delayed action risks perforation and sepsis. Acid suppression does not treat the underlying ischemic-infectious injury.
SubChapter: Gastrointestinal Complications

Q658. Answer: D

Explanation: A positive FTA-ABS confirms congenital syphilis, characterized by rhinitis, rash, and hepatosplenomegaly. A negative Coombs test rules out hemolytic disease, normal CSF VDRL excludes neurosyphilis, and elevated liver enzymes are nonspecific.
SubChapter: Infectious Complications

Q659. Answer: A

Explanation: Maternal hyperglycemia stimulates excess fetal insulin production; when the placental glucose supply ceases at birth, persistent hyperinsulinemia drives hypoglycemia. Liver immaturity and cortisol deficiency can contribute but are secondary factors.
SubChapter: Endocrine Complications

Q660. Answer: A

Explanation: Positive-pressure ventilation can rupture alveoli, trapping air in the pleural space under pressure that shifts the mediastinum and causes hypotension. Immediate decompression relieves distress. Pneumomediastinum produces subcutaneous crepitus, not severe hemodynamic compromise.
SubChapter: Cardiorespiratory Complications

Q661. Answer: A

Explanation: Meconium ileus, often associated with cystic fibrosis, results from viscid intestinal contents obstructing the ileum and producing microcolon. Hirschsprung disease shows a transition zone. Duodenal atresia gives a "double-bubble" image. Small-left-colon syndrome resolves spontaneously.
SubChapter: Gastrointestinal Complications

Q662. Answer: D

Explanation: Maternal IgG antibodies may cause transient neonatal thrombocytopenia; careful monitoring and selective transfusion prevent unnecessary intervention. Exchange transfusion or iron does not address immune destruction. Antibiotics are not indicated without infection signs.
SubChapter: Hematologic Complications

Q663. Answer: A

Explanation: Neonatal HSV infection with CNS involvement requires 21 days of IV acyclovir and repeat CSF PCR to confirm viral clearance. Topical or short oral therapy is inadequate. Antibiotics do not affect HSV replication.
SubChapter: Infectious Complications

Q664. Answer: A

Explanation: Beckwith-Wiedemann syndrome increases risk for embryonal tumors such as Wilms tumor and hepatoblastoma; periodic abdominal ultrasound and AFP monitoring during infancy are recommended. Cardiac, neurologic, or short-term glucose follow-up alone would miss tumor surveillance.
SubChapter: Genetic/Endocrine Complications

Q665. Answer: A

Explanation: Lung-protective ventilation and careful oxygen titration minimize barotrauma and oxidative injury, reducing bronchopulmonary dysplasia severity. Excessive PEEP or early corticosteroid use has adverse effects. Abrupt withdrawal of support causes hypoxia and acidosis.
SubChapter: Cardiorespiratory Complications

Q666. Answer: A

Explanation: Laryngomalacia, due to floppy supraglottic tissue, produces inspiratory stridor that worsens supine and improves prone. Tracheoesophageal fistula causes choking on feeds. Vocal-cord paralysis presents with weak cry and airway obstruction. Choanal atresia causes cyanosis relieved by crying.
SubChapter: Cardiorespiratory Complications

Q667. Answer: B

Explanation: Listeria monocytogenes causes late-onset neonatal meningitis, especially in preterm or immunocompromised infants, with characteristic CSF findings. Enteroviruses usually yield normal glucose. Staphylococcal and fungal infections are uncommon without risk factors like catheters or antibiotics.
SubChapter: Infectious Complications

Q668. Answer: A

Explanation: Neonatal abstinence syndrome is managed initially with nonpharmacologic measures—swaddling, quiet environment, and frequent feeds—to reduce withdrawal stress. Anticonvulsants and fluid restriction are inappropriate unless seizures or fluid overload occur.
SubChapter: Neurologic Complications

Q669. Answer: A

Explanation: Prostaglandin E1 keeps the ductus arteriosus open, allowing mixing between systemic and pulmonary circulations in ductal-dependent lesions like transposition. Diuretics or beta-blockers worsen perfusion. Pacing has no role.
SubChapter: Cardiorespiratory Complications

Q670. Answer: A

Explanation: Periventricular leukomalacia, a white-matter ischemic injury in preterm infants, commonly results in spastic cerebral palsy affecting lower extremities. Muscular dystrophy and congenital myasthenia are genetic neuromuscular disorders. Autism is multifactorial, not directly linked to this lesion.
SubChapter: Neurologic Complications
Q671. Answer: C
Explanation: TTN occurs from delayed clearance of lung fluid, common after cesarean birth. Symptoms include rapid breathing and mild distress that resolve within 48–72 hours. RDS appears earlier and more severe, meconium aspiration involves meconium staining, and pneumothorax causes sudden deterioration.
SubChapter: Respiratory Complications
Q672. Answer: A
Explanation: RDS results from surfactant deficiency leading to alveolar collapse and hypoxia, characterized radiographically by a ground-glass pattern. TTN resolves quickly, PPHN causes right-to-left shunting with loud murmurs, and pneumonia presents later with leukocytosis and infiltrates.
SubChapter: Respiratory Complications
Q673. Answer: A
Explanation: Meconium aspiration obstructs airways and causes chemical pneumonitis. Immediate oxygen and ventilatory support prevent hypoxemia. Stimulating crying increases aspiration risk, and antibiotics are secondary unless infection develops.
SubChapter: Respiratory Complications
Q674. Answer: A
Explanation: Choanal atresia obstructs posterior nasal passages, causing cyanosis during feeding that resolves when the mouth opens for crying. It requires airway maintenance and surgical correction. Other causes do not show this positional cyanosis pattern.
SubChapter: Congenital & Genetic Conditions
Q675. Answer: C
Explanation: Apnea of prematurity responds to gentle tactile stimulation to restart breathing. Persistent or frequent episodes may need caffeine therapy and cardiorespiratory monitoring. Immediate compressions are unnecessary unless apnea persists beyond 30 seconds.
SubChapter: Respiratory Complications
Q676. Answer: A
Explanation: For mild hypoglycemia (25–40 mg/dL) and asymptomatic or mildly symptomatic infants, early feeding provides rapid glucose correction. Persistent or severe cases require IV dextrose. Hypothermia worsens hypoglycemia but is not the primary treatment focus.
SubChapter: Metabolic & Hematologic Disorders
Q677. Answer: A
Explanation: Fetomaternal hemorrhage causes acute neonatal anemia from placental blood loss into the maternal circulation, leading to pallor and tachycardia. Polycythemia presents with ruddy color and sluggish perfusion; hypoglycemia causes jitteriness; hyperbilirubinemia appears later.
SubChapter: Metabolic & Hematologic Disorders
Q678. Answer: A
Explanation: Bilirubin of 16 mg/dL at 48 hours indicates significant hyperbilirubinemia requiring phototherapy to prevent kernicterus. Phototherapy promotes bilirubin breakdown and excretion. Observation alone is unsafe at this level, and window sunlight is ineffective and potentially harmful.
SubChapter: Metabolic & Hematologic Disorders
Q679. Answer: D

Explanation: These nonspecific symptoms suggest neonatal sepsis. Blood culture identifies the causative organism for targeted antibiotic therapy. CBC aids assessment but cannot confirm infection alone; glucose and bilirubin evaluate other metabolic issues.
SubChapter: Infectious Conditions
Q680. Answer: A
Explanation: Neonatal sepsis due to maternal chorioamnionitis requires immediate empiric IV antibiotics after obtaining cultures to prevent rapid progression to septic shock. Observation or waiting for labs risks deterioration. Thermal support is secondary to infection control.
SubChapter: Infectious Conditions
Q681. Answer: A
Explanation: Hypoxic-ischemic encephalopathy results from perinatal asphyxia, causing seizures and neurologic depression. Intraventricular hemorrhage may coexist but usually presents with bulging fontanel and apnea. Hypoglycemia causes jitteriness, not tonic seizures; alkalosis is metabolic, not neurologic.
SubChapter: Neurologic & Thermoregulatory Disorders
Q682. Answer: A
Explanation: Hypothermia reduces metabolic efficiency and oxygenation in neonates, leading to acidosis and hypoglycemia. Prompt rewarming using a radiant warmer restores temperature balance. Feeding and infection assessment follow stabilization but are not initial interventions.
SubChapter: Neurologic & Thermoregulatory Disorders
Q683. Answer: D
Explanation: PPHN occurs when pulmonary vascular resistance remains high after birth, maintaining fetal circulation patterns with right-to-left shunting. Oxygen therapy is often ineffective. Structural defects such as VSD or PDA present differently and often with less severe cyanosis.
SubChapter: Respiratory Complications
Q684. Answer: A
Explanation: Congenital CMV causes multisystem involvement including jaundice, hepatosplenomegaly, and neurologic damage. It results from maternal viral transmission during pregnancy. Toxoplasmosis presents similarly but is linked to cat exposure; erythroblastosis causes anemia, not viral inclusion bodies.
SubChapter: Infectious Conditions
Q685. Answer: A
Explanation: Neonatal abstinence syndrome results from withdrawal after in-utero opioid exposure. Treatment includes pharmacologic therapy (e.g., morphine titration) and environmental control to minimize stimuli. Early intervention prevents dehydration, seizures, and growth failure.
SubChapter: Neurologic & Thermoregulatory Disorders
Q686. Answer: A
Explanation: Hematocrit above 65% indicates neonatal polycythemia, which increases blood viscosity and impairs perfusion. Partial exchange transfusion with saline reduces viscosity and prevents complications like stroke or necrotizing enterocolitis. Phototherapy treats bilirubin, not polycythemia.
SubChapter: Metabolic & Hematologic Disorders
Q687. Answer: C
Explanation: Premature infants lose heat quickly due to low brown fat and thin skin. Maintaining a neutral thermal environment prevents cold stress, which increases oxygen and glucose use, risking acidosis. Other interventions follow stabilization.
SubChapter: Neurologic & Thermoregulatory Disorders
Q688. Answer: A

Explanation: PDA produces continuous "machinery" murmur and bounding pulses from left-to-right shunting. VSD causes holosystolic murmur; coarctation leads to weak femoral pulses; Tetralogy produces cyanotic spells rather than bounding pulses.
SubChapter: Congenital & Genetic Conditions
Q689. Answer: A
Explanation: Erb's palsy results from brachial plexus injury (C5–C6) during shoulder dystocia, producing "waiter's tip" posture with limp upper arm but preserved grip. Klumpke's affects hand function, phrenic causes respiratory distress, and facial nerve palsy affects facial symmetry.
SubChapter: Neurologic & Thermoregulatory Disorders
Q690. Answer: A
Explanation: Early-onset GBS sepsis presents within 24–48 hours with respiratory distress, temperature instability, and feeding difficulty. Rapid antibiotic therapy is essential to prevent shock and meningitis. Late-onset sepsis appears after one week and is typically nosocomial.
SubChapter: Infectious Conditions
Q691. Answer: D
Explanation: Apnea of prematurity is due to immature respiratory control. Initial nursing management includes gentle tactile stimulation and airway clearance to reinitiate breathing. Caffeine therapy and cardiorespiratory monitoring are considered after stabilization. Immediate compressions are unnecessary unless apnea persists beyond 30 seconds.
SubChapter: Respiratory Complications
Q692. Answer: A
Explanation: Sudden asymmetrical chest movement and decreased breath sounds suggest pneumothorax, often due to barotrauma from mechanical ventilation. Rapid assessment and possible needle decompression are essential. RDS and BPD cause diffuse distress, not unilateral findings, while atelectasis develops gradually.
SubChapter: Respiratory Complications
Q693. Answer: A
Explanation: Tetralogy of Fallot combines four heart defects causing right-to-left shunt and cyanosis unrelieved by oxygen. The boot-shaped cardiac silhouette on imaging is characteristic. VSD and PDA produce left-to-right shunts, while coarctation causes differential pulses without generalized cyanosis.
SubChapter: Congenital & Genetic Conditions
Q694. Answer: A
Explanation: Severe hypoglycemia (<25 mg/dL) requires IV dextrose to prevent neurologic injury. Early feeding treats mild cases, but this value demands prompt IV correction. Hypothermia management is secondary once glucose levels stabilize. Continuous glucose monitoring follows treatment initiation.
SubChapter: Metabolic & Hematologic Disorders
Q695. Answer: C
Explanation: Hemolytic disease from Rh incompatibility may require exchange transfusion to remove sensitized red cells and reduce bilirubin toxicity. Phototherapy alone is inadequate for severe hemolysis. IV fluids support perfusion but do not remove antibodies. Iron is given later for recovery.
SubChapter: Metabolic & Hematologic Disorders
Q696. Answer: A
Explanation: Early-onset GBS sepsis is a medical emergency requiring immediate empiric IV antibiotics after cultures. Delay in therapy greatly increases mortality risk. Supportive care, including temperature control, follows antibiotic initiation but should not precede it.
SubChapter: Infectious Conditions
Q697. Answer: A

Explanation: Neonatal abstinence syndrome arises from in-utero opioid exposure, causing withdrawal signs such as irritability, tremors, and abnormal sleep. Management includes pharmacologic therapy and environmental modifications. Hypoglycemia may cause jitteriness but lacks yawning or irritability.
SubChapter: Neurologic & Thermoregulatory Disorders

Q698. Answer: A

Explanation: Biliary atresia causes obstructed bile flow, resulting in conjugated hyperbilirubinemia, pale stools, and dark urine. Unlike physiologic or breast milk jaundice, it requires surgical correction to prevent liver failure. Hemolytic anemia produces unconjugated jaundice without pale stool.
SubChapter: Metabolic & Hematologic Disorders

Q699. Answer: D

Explanation: Cold stress increases oxygen consumption and anaerobic metabolism, causing metabolic acidosis and hypoglycemia. Immediate rewarming and glucose monitoring are required. Sepsis may present similarly but usually includes temperature instability with other systemic signs.
SubChapter: Neurologic & Thermoregulatory Disorders

Q700. Answer: A

Explanation: Infants with AV canal defect have increased pulmonary flow and heart failure risk. Nursing care includes controlled feeding with frequent rest and fluid balance monitoring. Early cardiology involvement ensures timely surgical repair. Overfeeding or delayed management worsens cardiac strain.
SubChapter: Congenital & Genetic Conditions

Questions (701-750)

Q701. A 30-week premature infant develops grunting, nasal flaring, and intercostal retractions shortly after birth. Chest X-ray shows "ground-glass" opacity. Which treatment should the nurse anticipate?

A. Surfactant replacement therapy
B. Broad-spectrum antibiotics
C. Exchange transfusion
D. Phototherapy

Q702. A term newborn develops cyanosis and tachypnea unresponsive to oxygen. Echocardiogram shows pulmonary vascular resistance higher than systemic pressure. What is the diagnosis?

A. Persistent pulmonary hypertension of the newborn (PPHN)
B. Transient tachypnea of the newborn
C. Meconium aspiration
D. Ventricular septal defect

Q703. A neonate is jittery, has a weak cry, and blood glucose of 35 mg/dL. The infant was born to a diabetic mother. What is the immediate nursing action?

A. Delay feeding until warmer
B. Observe and repeat glucose later
C. Administer insulin
D. Feed the infant or give glucose gel

Q704. A newborn presents with severe jaundice within 12 hours of birth, pallor, and hepatosplenomegaly. Maternal blood type is O negative; infant is O positive. What is the likely diagnosis?

A. Hemolytic disease due to Rh incompatibility
B. Physiologic jaundice
C. Breast milk jaundice
D. Biliary atresia

Q705. A newborn delivered after prolonged rupture of membranes has temperature instability, lethargy, and poor feeding. Which diagnostic test should be obtained first?

A. Blood culture
B. Serum bilirubin
C. Cranial ultrasound
D. Arterial blood gas

Q706. A 2-day-old newborn on mechanical ventilation becomes suddenly cyanotic with unequal breath sounds and a deviated trachea. What should the nurse suspect?

A. Tension pneumothorax
B. Bronchopulmonary dysplasia
C. Meconium aspiration
D. Persistent pulmonary hypertension

Q707. A neonate is cyanotic when crying improves oxygenation, but cyanosis worsens when quiet. What congenital defect is indicated?

A. Pulmonary atresia
B. Tetralogy of Fallot
C. Coarctation of the aorta
D. Choanal atresia

Q708. A newborn exhibits poor feeding, hypotonia, and tremors after maternal cocaine use during pregnancy. What should the nurse anticipate?

A. Neonatal withdrawal management with supportive care

B. Phototherapy
C. Exchange transfusion
D. Immediate antibiotic therapy

Q709. A neonate with cleft palate has difficulty coordinating sucking and swallowing. What is the nurse's best action?
A. Use a specialized feeder with slow-flow nipple
B. Attempt breastfeeding in side-lying position
C. Insert nasogastric tube immediately
D. Delay feeding until surgical repair

Q710. A full-term infant develops irritability, high-pitched cry, and poor feeding at 24 hours. Mother is positive for syphilis. Which diagnostic test confirms the condition?
A. VDRL or RPR test on infant serum
B. TORCH antibody screening
C. Cerebrospinal fluid culture only
D. Blood glucose measurement

Q711. A preterm newborn develops oxygen dependence and recurrent wheezing after prolonged ventilation for RDS. Chest X-ray reveals hyperinflation and areas of atelectasis. What condition should the nurse suspect?
A. Persistent pulmonary hypertension
B. Pneumothorax
C. Meconium aspiration syndrome
D. Bronchopulmonary dysplasia (BPD)

Q712. A newborn delivered at 29 weeks gestation develops pallor, hypotension, bulging fontanel, and apnea. What complication is most likely?
A. Intraventricular hemorrhage (IVH)
B. Hypoglycemia
C. Sepsis
D. RDS

Q713. A neonate presents with severe respiratory distress immediately after birth and scaphoid abdomen. Breath sounds are diminished on the left. What is the likely diagnosis?
A. Congenital diaphragmatic hernia
B. Pneumothorax
C. Tracheoesophageal fistula
D. Pulmonary hypoplasia

Q714. A 2-day-old infant exhibits irritability, tremors, diarrhea, and poor feeding. The mother used opioids during pregnancy. What nursing intervention is appropriate?
A. Decrease environmental stimuli and provide gentle swaddling
B. Encourage frequent handling for comfort
C. Administer IV glucose for energy
D. Avoid pharmacologic treatment unless seizures occur

Q715. A term newborn exhibits jaundice, irritability, and muscle rigidity on day four of life. Total bilirubin level is 28 mg/dL. What complication has likely occurred?
A. Biliary atresia
B. Physiologic jaundice
C. Kernicterus
D. Sepsis

Q716. A preterm infant on mechanical ventilation shows sudden cyanosis, bradycardia, and diminished right-sided breath sounds. What should the nurse do first?

A. Notify provider and prepare for needle decompression
B. Increase oxygen flow
C. Suction airway for mucus
D. Adjust ventilator settings

Q717. A neonate born at 28 weeks gestation has weak cry, lethargy, and temperature 35.2°C (95.3°F). What is the primary nursing goal?

A. Prevent cold stress through thermal regulation
B. Begin IV fluids immediately
C. Administer antibiotics prophylactically
D. Stimulate frequent crying

Q718. A newborn develops tachypnea, grunting, and nasal flaring six hours after cesarean birth. Symptoms improve after 48 hours. What diagnosis fits this pattern?

A. Transient tachypnea of the newborn (TTN)
B. Respiratory distress syndrome
C. Meconium aspiration
D. Pneumonia

Q719. A 3-day-old term infant has hypothermia, lethargy, poor feeding, and hypotension. Mother had prolonged rupture of membranes. Which infection is most likely?

A. Cytomegalovirus
B. Late-onset sepsis
C. Meningitis only
D. Early-onset neonatal sepsis

Q720. A newborn presents with cyanosis that worsens during crying and improves with squatting. What congenital condition does this pattern suggest?

A. Tetralogy of Fallot
B. Transposition of great arteries
C. Tricuspid atresia
D. Patent ductus arteriosus

Q721. A 33-week preterm infant develops tachypnea, nasal flaring, and retractions 20 minutes after birth. Surfactant therapy is initiated, but oxygen demand remains high. What additional intervention should the nurse anticipate?

A. Continuous positive airway pressure (CPAP)
B. Chest physiotherapy
C. Diuretic therapy
D. Oral feeding initiation

Q722. A full-term infant presents with irritability, jaundice, and total serum bilirubin of 22 mg/dL on day three. Which treatment should the nurse prepare for?

A. Intensive phototherapy
B. Exchange transfusion
C. Observation only
D. Intravenous antibiotics

Q723. A neonate of a mother with poorly controlled diabetes shows tremors, irritability, and blood glucose of 32 mg/dL. What is the best initial nursing action?

A. Keep the infant NPO for 6 hours
B. Begin IV insulin therapy
C. Monitor glucose without intervention
D. Feed the infant or administer glucose gel

Q724. A neonate develops cyanosis within minutes of birth, which does not improve with oxygen. Echocardiogram shows aorta arising from the right ventricle and pulmonary artery from the left ventricle. What is the diagnosis?

A. Transposition of the great arteries (TGA)
B. Tetralogy of Fallot
C. Patent ductus arteriosus
D. Truncus arteriosus

Q725. A 2-day-old infant exhibits fever, poor feeding, and respiratory distress. Maternal history reveals untreated Group B Streptococcus colonization. What is the priority nursing action?

A. Obtain cultures and initiate IV antibiotics
B. Increase fluids and observe
C. Delay treatment until lab confirmation
D. Place under warmer only

Q726. A preterm infant at 29 weeks has oxygen dependence and recurrent wheezing. Chest X-ray shows cystic changes and hyperinflation. What chronic complication has developed?

A. Bronchopulmonary dysplasia (BPD)
B. Pulmonary edema
C. Pneumothorax
D. Transient tachypnea

Q727. A neonate displays hypothermia, pallor, and weak cry in a cool delivery room. Which nursing intervention has the highest priority?

A. Apply cold compresses to head
B. Provide oral feeding for energy
C. Massage extremities to improve circulation
D. Rewarm using a radiant warmer and monitor temperature

Q728. A 36-hour-old infant exhibits excessive sleepiness, poor feeding, and high-pitched cry. Total bilirubin is 18 mg/dL. Which complication is the nurse most concerned about?

A. Bilirubin encephalopathy
B. Sepsis
C. Metabolic acidosis
D. Dehydration

Q729. A 1-day-old newborn with cleft lip is unable to maintain suction during feeding. What should the nurse recommend to the parents?

A. Use a specialized feeder with compressible reservoir
B. Attempt breastfeeding only in side-lying position
C. Insert nasogastric tube routinely
D. Delay feeding until surgical repair

Q730. A preterm infant born at 30 weeks develops abdominal distension, bloody stools, and bilious vomiting. X-ray shows pneumatosis intestinalis. What condition is suspected?

A. Necrotizing enterocolitis (NEC)
B. Hirschsprung disease
C. Intestinal atresia
D. Pyloric stenosis

Q731. A 2-day-old preterm infant develops abdominal distension, bloody stools, and gastric residuals with a "soap-bubble" appearance on X-ray. What condition is suspected?

A. Necrotizing enterocolitis (NEC)
B. Hirschsprung disease
C. Meconium ileus

D. Gastroesophageal reflux

Q732. A newborn of a diabetic mother exhibits respiratory distress shortly after birth. Blood glucose is 48 mg/dL, and chest X-ray shows reticulogranular infiltrates. What complication is most likely?

A. Bronchopulmonary dysplasia

B. Transient tachypnea of the newborn

C. Meconium aspiration

D. Respiratory distress syndrome (RDS)

Q733. A 3-day-old infant presents with irritability, jaundice, and dark urine. Laboratory findings reveal conjugated bilirubin elevation. What condition should the nurse suspect?

A. Biliary atresia

B. Physiologic jaundice

C. Hemolytic anemia

D. Breast milk jaundice

Q734. A preterm infant suddenly develops apnea, bradycardia, and bulging fontanel. What should the nurse suspect?

A. Intraventricular hemorrhage (IVH)

B. Hypoglycemia

C. Sepsis

D. Anemia

Q735. A term infant presents with persistent tachypnea, grunting, and intercostal retractions six hours after cesarean birth. The symptoms resolve within 48 hours. What is the likely diagnosis?

A. Transient tachypnea of the newborn (TTN)

B. Respiratory distress syndrome

C. Pneumonia

D. Persistent pulmonary hypertension

Q736. A newborn with Down syndrome presents with poor feeding, tachypnea, and cyanosis. Echocardiography confirms atrioventricular septal defect. What is the nurse's priority intervention?

A. Delay follow-up until six months

B. Encourage vigorous oral feeding to increase intake

C. Restrict fluids completely

D. Support nutrition with small, frequent feedings

Q737. A 1-day-old neonate becomes lethargic, with poor feeding and temperature instability. Blood culture confirms E. coli. What is the priority nursing goal?

A. Prevent septic shock through early antibiotic administration

B. Provide continuous enteral nutrition

C. Maintain NPO status for 48 hours

D. Delay treatment until WBC results return

Q738. A premature infant on ventilator support shows sudden desaturation, asymmetric chest rise, and diminished left breath sounds. What is the likely cause?

A. Pneumothorax

B. Bronchopulmonary dysplasia

C. Pulmonary edema

D. Respiratory distress syndrome

Q739. A 38-week infant delivered after prolonged rupture of membranes has fever, lethargy, and poor feeding at 12 hours. Which infection is most likely?

A. Group B Streptococcus sepsis

B. Cytomegalovirus

C. Late-onset sepsis

D. Hepatitis B

Q740. A term newborn exhibits high-pitched cry, poor feeding, and hypertonia 48 hours after birth. Maternal history includes untreated syphilis. What diagnostic test confirms this condition?

A. Urinalysis
B. TORCH screen only
C. Blood glucose measurement
D. VDRL or RPR on infant serum

Q741. A 2-day-old preterm infant develops sudden abdominal distension, bloody stools, and visible bowel loops. X-ray shows pneumatosis intestinalis. What is the first nursing action?

A. Stop all oral feedings and notify provider
B. Increase feeding volume for bowel motility
C. Administer glycerin suppository
D. Apply warm compress to abdomen

Q742. A term infant born after a prolonged, difficult labor exhibits pallor, tachycardia, and hematocrit of 25%. Which cause is most likely?

A. Fetomaternal hemorrhage
B. Polycythemia
C. Dehydration
D. Sepsis

Q743. A 35-week infant on oxygen therapy exhibits chronic tachypnea, retractions, and X-ray findings of hyperinflated lungs with fibrosis. What long-term condition is indicated?

A. Bronchopulmonary dysplasia (BPD)
B. Transient tachypnea of the newborn
C. Pneumothorax
D. Meconium aspiration syndrome

Q744. A 38-week infant exhibits generalized cyanosis that worsens with crying and is unresponsive to oxygen. Cardiac imaging reveals overriding aorta and right ventricular hypertrophy. What diagnosis is confirmed?

A. Tricuspid atresia
B. Transposition of the great arteries
C. Pulmonary stenosis
D. Tetralogy of Fallot

Q745. A newborn delivered via cesarean exhibits rapid respirations (80/min) and mild retractions but no cyanosis. Symptoms improve within 48 hours. What is the likely cause?

A. Transient tachypnea of the newborn (TTN)
B. Respiratory distress syndrome
C. Aspiration pneumonia
D. Persistent pulmonary hypertension

Q746. A neonate is jittery, irritable, and has blood glucose of 28 mg/dL. Which action should the nurse take first?

A. Feed the infant immediately with formula or breast milk
B. Administer IV insulin to stabilize glucose
C. Recheck glucose in one hour
D. Place under radiant warmer and monitor

Q747. A 30-week preterm infant exhibits poor muscle tone, weak cry, and temperature of 35.0°C (95°F). What is the nurse's first intervention?

A. Place the infant in a preheated incubator
B. Offer oral glucose water

C. Provide vigorous tactile stimulation
D. Begin antibiotic therapy

Q748. A 3-day-old infant displays vomiting, poor feeding, and metabolic acidosis. Urinalysis reveals elevated ketones and maple syrup odor. What metabolic disorder is suspected?

A. Hypothyroidism
B. Phenylketonuria
C. Galactosemia
D. Maple syrup urine disease

Q749. A newborn presents with irritability, high-pitched cry, and tremors. The mother used opioids during pregnancy. What nursing intervention is most appropriate?

A. Decrease stimuli, swaddle tightly, and maintain calm environment
B. Encourage frequent handling for bonding
C. Restrict feeding to prevent vomiting
D. Begin phototherapy for hyperbilirubinemia

Q750. A 4-day-old term infant has persistent jaundice, pale stools, and dark urine. Laboratory results show conjugated hyperbilirubinemia. What condition should the nurse suspect?

A. Biliary atresia
B. Physiologic jaundice
C. Breast milk jaundice
D. Hemolytic anemia

Answer key and Explanation (701-750)

Q701. Answer: A

Explanation: Premature infants often develop respiratory distress syndrome from surfactant deficiency. Surfactant administration improves alveolar expansion and oxygenation. Antibiotics are used for infection; transfusion and phototherapy address hematologic or bilirubin issues, not respiratory immaturity.

SubChapter: Respiratory Complications

Q702. Answer: A

Explanation: PPHN occurs when fetal circulation persists after birth due to elevated pulmonary pressure, causing right-to-left shunting and severe hypoxemia unrelieved by oxygen. It differs from TTN, which resolves spontaneously, and from structural cardiac defects such as VSD.

SubChapter: Respiratory Complications

Q703. Answer: D

Explanation: Infants of diabetic mothers experience hypoglycemia from hyperinsulinemia. Early feeding or glucose gel rapidly raises blood sugar and prevents neurologic injury. Insulin worsens hypoglycemia, and delaying feeding increases risk of seizures.

SubChapter: Metabolic & Hematologic Disorders

Q704. Answer: A

Explanation: Early-onset jaundice, anemia, and hepatosplenomegaly indicate Rh hemolytic disease. Maternal antibodies destroy fetal red cells, causing hyperbilirubinemia. Physiologic jaundice occurs later and milder; biliary atresia presents weeks later with cholestasis.

SubChapter: Metabolic & Hematologic Disorders

Q705. Answer: A

Explanation: These nonspecific symptoms suggest neonatal sepsis. Blood cultures identify pathogens before starting empiric antibiotics. Delay increases mortality risk. Bilirubin and ABG help evaluate other systems, but infection confirmation is the priority.

SubChapter: Infectious Conditions

Q706. Answer: A

Explanation: Sudden desaturation with asymmetric chest movement and tracheal deviation suggests tension pneumothorax. Immediate decompression is required to relieve intrathoracic pressure. BPD and PPHN are chronic conditions; meconium aspiration causes coarse crackles without tracheal shift.

SubChapter: Respiratory Complications

Q707. Answer: D

Explanation: Choanal atresia causes nasal airway obstruction, leading to cyanosis during quiet periods that resolves with crying when oral breathing begins. It requires airway maintenance and surgical correction. Cardiac defects cause persistent, not positional, cyanosis.

SubChapter: Congenital & Genetic Conditions

Q708. Answer: A

Explanation: Infants exposed to stimulants like cocaine often show withdrawal symptoms including irritability and tremors. Supportive care involves minimizing stimulation and monitoring feeding. Antibiotics and transfusion are unrelated; phototherapy treats hyperbilirubinemia, not drug withdrawal.

SubChapter: Neurologic & Thermoregulatory Disorders

Q709. Answer: A

Explanation: Specialized cleft feeders allow milk flow control, enabling effective nutrition without aspiration. Breastfeeding is often ineffective until repair, and tube feeding is reserved for severe aspiration risk. Early intervention promotes growth before surgical correction.

SubChapter: Congenital & Genetic Conditions

Q710. Answer: A
Explanation: Venereal Disease Research Laboratory (VDRL) or Rapid Plasma Reagin (RPR) tests detect syphilis antibodies in infant serum, confirming congenital infection. TORCH screening is broader and nonspecific; CSF culture evaluates CNS infection; glucose measures metabolic status, not infection.
SubChapter: Infectious Conditions

Q711. Answer: D
Explanation: BPD is a chronic lung condition from prolonged oxygen and ventilator exposure, leading to inflammation, fibrosis, and uneven aeration. Pneumothorax causes acute deterioration; meconium aspiration occurs in term infants; PPHN presents at birth with severe hypoxemia.
SubChapter: Respiratory Complications

Q712. Answer: A
Explanation: IVH results from fragile cerebral vessels in preterm infants, often triggered by hypoxia or rapid volume changes. Symptoms include bulging fontanel, apnea, and pallor. RDS affects breathing mechanics, while hypoglycemia and sepsis cause metabolic or systemic signs, not increased intracranial pressure.
SubChapter: Neurologic & Thermoregulatory Disorders

Q713. Answer: A
Explanation: A scaphoid abdomen with respiratory distress indicates congenital diaphragmatic hernia, where abdominal organs herniate into the thorax, compressing lungs. Immediate respiratory support and surgical correction are critical. Pneumothorax and TEF present differently, while hypoplasia is often secondary.
SubChapter: Congenital & Genetic Conditions

Q714. Answer: A
Explanation: Neonatal abstinence syndrome requires minimizing stimuli, swaddling, and sometimes pharmacologic therapy to reduce withdrawal symptoms. Excessive handling worsens irritability. Glucose does not address withdrawal, and delayed treatment risks complications like dehydration or seizures.
SubChapter: Neurologic & Thermoregulatory Disorders

Q715. Answer: C
Explanation: Kernicterus is bilirubin-induced neurologic dysfunction due to extremely high unconjugated bilirubin crossing the blood–brain barrier, causing irreversible brain injury. Physiologic jaundice is mild; biliary atresia is cholestatic; sepsis presents with temperature instability and poor perfusion.
SubChapter: Metabolic & Hematologic Disorders

Q716. Answer: A
Explanation: These findings indicate tension pneumothorax, a medical emergency requiring decompression to restore lung expansion. Increasing oxygen or suctioning will not relieve the pressure. Prompt intervention prevents cardiac arrest from mediastinal shift.
SubChapter: Respiratory Complications

Q717. Answer: A
Explanation: Preterm infants lack brown fat and have immature thermoregulation, making them prone to hypothermia. Maintaining a neutral thermal environment minimizes oxygen and glucose consumption, preventing metabolic acidosis. IV fluids and antibiotics are secondary after temperature stabilization.
SubChapter: Neurologic & Thermoregulatory Disorders

Q718. Answer: A
Explanation: TTN results from delayed clearance of fetal lung fluid, particularly in cesarean deliveries. It resolves within 2–3 days without long-term effects. RDS presents earlier and more severe; meconium aspiration affects term/post-term infants; pneumonia develops later.
SubChapter: Respiratory Complications

Q719. Answer: D

Explanation: Early-onset sepsis, often from Group B Streptococcus or E. coli, presents within 72 hours after birth. Symptoms include temperature instability, lethargy, and cardiovascular compromise. Late-onset sepsis occurs after the first week and often originates from hospital exposure.

SubChapter: Infectious Conditions

Q720. Answer: A

Explanation: "Tet spells," characterized by cyanosis during crying and relief with squatting, are typical of Tetralogy of Fallot. Squatting increases systemic vascular resistance, reducing right-to-left shunting. Transposition causes constant cyanosis, while PDA produces bounding pulses rather than cyanotic episodes.

SubChapter: Congenital & Genetic Conditions

Q721. Answer: A

Explanation: CPAP provides consistent airway pressure to maintain alveolar expansion and improve oxygenation in respiratory distress syndrome. It complements surfactant therapy. Chest physiotherapy is not used acutely in neonates, diuretics are for chronic conditions, and feeding is withheld during respiratory compromise.

SubChapter: Respiratory Complications

Q722. Answer: A

Explanation: Phototherapy is indicated for moderate to severe hyperbilirubinemia in term infants, reducing unconjugated bilirubin through photo-oxidation. Exchange transfusion is reserved for dangerously high or unresponsive cases. Observation alone risks kernicterus, and antibiotics are not indicated unless infection is suspected.

SubChapter: Metabolic & Hematologic Disorders

Q723. Answer: D

Explanation: Hypoglycemia in infants of diabetic mothers is treated promptly with oral feeding or glucose gel to prevent seizures and brain injury. Insulin is contraindicated, and withholding feeds worsens hypoglycemia. Monitoring follows treatment to assess stability.

SubChapter: Metabolic & Hematologic Disorders

Q724. Answer: A

Explanation: TGA causes parallel circulation with no oxygen exchange between systemic and pulmonary circuits. Cyanosis persists despite oxygen therapy. Maintaining ductal patency with prostaglandin E1 allows mixing until surgical correction. Other defects present with different shunt patterns or murmurs.

SubChapter: Congenital & Genetic Conditions

Q725. Answer: A

Explanation: Early-onset neonatal sepsis, often due to GBS, requires immediate empiric antibiotic therapy after blood cultures. Delay increases morbidity and mortality. Supportive care follows antibiotic initiation. Observation or warming alone does not address infection.

SubChapter: Infectious Conditions

Q726. Answer: A

Explanation: BPD results from prolonged oxygen and ventilator exposure leading to lung injury, fibrosis, and chronic respiratory symptoms. It is managed with oxygen titration, fluid restriction, and nutritional support. Pneumothorax and TTN are acute, while pulmonary edema is secondary to cardiac or renal causes.

SubChapter: Respiratory Complications

Q727. Answer: D

Explanation: Hypothermia causes increased oxygen consumption and metabolic acidosis in newborns. Gradual rewarming under a radiant warmer restores thermoregulation and prevents complications. Feeding and stimulation are delayed until stable temperature and perfusion are achieved.

SubChapter: Neurologic & Thermoregulatory Disorders

Q728. Answer: A

Explanation: Neurologic symptoms at high bilirubin levels suggest bilirubin encephalopathy (kernicterus). Immediate intensive phototherapy and possibly exchange transfusion are required to prevent permanent brain injury. Sepsis may mimic these signs but typically includes temperature instability and hypotension.

SubChapter: Metabolic & Hematologic Disorders

Q729. Answer: A

Explanation: Specialized feeders like Haberman bottles allow milk flow control and compensate for suction deficits. They promote adequate nutrition and prevent aspiration before surgical repair. Tube feeding is reserved for severe cases or associated airway compromise.

SubChapter: Congenital & Genetic Conditions

Q730. Answer: A

Explanation: NEC is a severe gastrointestinal emergency in preterm infants due to ischemic and bacterial injury. Findings include distension, bloody stools, and gas in bowel walls (pneumatosis). Immediate cessation of feeds, gastric decompression, and antibiotics are essential.

SubChapter: Infectious Conditions

Q731. Answer: A

Explanation: NEC is a life-threatening intestinal disorder in preterm infants caused by ischemic and bacterial injury. The hallmark radiographic sign is pneumatosis intestinalis, or gas within the bowel wall. Hirschsprung causes delayed meconium, and meconium ileus is related to cystic fibrosis.

SubChapter: Infectious Conditions

Q732. Answer: D

Explanation: Infants of diabetic mothers are at risk for delayed surfactant production leading to RDS, even at term. The reticulogranular "ground-glass" appearance on imaging confirms this diagnosis. TTN resolves faster; meconium aspiration causes coarse infiltrates; BPD is a chronic sequela of prolonged ventilation.

SubChapter: Respiratory Complications

Q733. Answer: A

Explanation: Biliary atresia causes conjugated hyperbilirubinemia due to obstruction of bile ducts, leading to dark urine, pale stools, and progressive liver failure. Physiologic and breast milk jaundice involve unconjugated bilirubin, and hemolytic anemia presents with anemia and unconjugated bilirubin rise.

SubChapter: Metabolic & Hematologic Disorders

Q734. Answer: A

Explanation: IVH is common in very low-birth-weight infants due to fragile cerebral vessels. Signs include apnea, hypotonia, and bulging fontanel from intracranial bleeding. Hypoglycemia causes jitteriness, sepsis produces temperature instability, and anemia develops gradually without acute neurologic signs.

SubChapter: Neurologic & Thermoregulatory Disorders

Q735. Answer: A

Explanation: TTN results from delayed lung fluid clearance, particularly after cesarean delivery. It causes mild respiratory distress that improves within two days. RDS is due to surfactant deficiency and lasts longer, while pneumonia or PPHN presents with systemic illness or severe hypoxia.

SubChapter: Respiratory Complications

Q736. Answer: D

Explanation: Infants with AV septal defects have increased pulmonary blood flow, causing fatigue and poor feeding. Small, frequent feeds conserve energy while meeting caloric needs. Overfeeding or fluid restriction can worsen failure symptoms. Early cardiology follow-up is essential.

SubChapter: Congenital & Genetic Conditions

Q737. Answer: A

Explanation: Early-onset E. coli sepsis can rapidly progress to shock. Immediate broad-spectrum antibiotics and supportive care stabilize perfusion and prevent multi-organ failure. Nutritional support follows stabilization. Delaying treatment for labs endangers the infant's life.

SubChapter: Infectious Conditions

Q738. Answer: A

Explanation: Sudden desaturation and unequal chest expansion indicate pneumothorax, often from positive pressure ventilation. Immediate decompression restores lung expansion. BPD and RDS cause bilateral distress, and pulmonary edema presents with crackles, not asymmetry.

SubChapter: Respiratory Complications

Q739. Answer: A

Explanation: Early-onset Group B Streptococcus sepsis occurs within 24 hours, presenting with respiratory distress, temperature instability, and lethargy. Cytomegalovirus causes congenital infection, and late-onset sepsis develops after one week. Prompt antibiotics are critical.

SubChapter: Infectious Conditions

Q740. Answer: D

Explanation: Congenital syphilis is confirmed through non-treponemal tests like VDRL or RPR on neonatal serum. It presents with irritability, hepatosplenomegaly, and rash. TORCH screening is general, and metabolic tests do not detect spirochete infection.

SubChapter: Infectious Conditions

Q741. Answer: A

Explanation: These findings confirm necrotizing enterocolitis, a gastrointestinal emergency. Immediate cessation of enteral feeds prevents further bowel perforation, while notifying the provider for antibiotics and decompression is critical. Increasing feeding or stimulation worsens bowel injury and raises mortality risk.

SubChapter: Infectious Conditions

Q742. Answer: A

Explanation: Fetomaternal hemorrhage occurs when fetal blood enters maternal circulation, leading to neonatal anemia with pallor and tachycardia. Polycythemia causes ruddy color; dehydration causes weight loss; sepsis may lower hematocrit later but initially shows temperature instability.

SubChapter: Metabolic & Hematologic Disorders

Q743. Answer: A

Explanation: BPD results from prolonged ventilator and oxygen exposure, causing alveolar damage, fibrosis, and chronic respiratory insufficiency. TTN resolves within 72 hours; pneumothorax presents suddenly; meconium aspiration affects term infants, not preterm ventilated babies.

SubChapter: Respiratory Complications

Q744. Answer: D

Explanation: Tetralogy of Fallot includes four defects leading to right-to-left shunting and cyanosis unrelieved by oxygen. The classic features—overriding aorta and right ventricular hypertrophy—differentiate it from transposition and other structural anomalies.

SubChapter: Congenital & Genetic Conditions

Q745. Answer: A

Explanation: TTN occurs from delayed fetal lung fluid clearance, especially after cesarean delivery. Symptoms are mild and self-limiting. RDS involves surfactant deficiency and severe hypoxia, while PPHN causes persistent cyanosis. Pneumonia appears later with infection signs.

SubChapter: Respiratory Complications

Q746. Answer: A

Explanation: Hypoglycemia below 30 mg/dL requires prompt oral feeding to restore glucose and prevent seizures or brain injury. IV glucose follows if symptoms persist. Insulin would worsen hypoglycemia, and waiting an hour risks neurologic damage.
SubChapter: Metabolic & Hematologic Disorders

Q747. Answer: A

Explanation: Hypothermia in preterm infants rapidly leads to metabolic acidosis and hypoglycemia. Maintaining neutral thermal environment via incubator prevents cold stress and physiologic deterioration. Glucose and antibiotics may follow if metabolic or infectious causes are confirmed.
SubChapter: Neurologic & Thermoregulatory Disorders

Q748. Answer: D

Explanation: Maple syrup urine disease involves defective branched-chain amino acid metabolism, causing ketoacidosis and characteristic sweet odor. Early recognition and dietary management prevent neurologic injury. PKU lacks acidosis; galactosemia presents with liver failure; hypothyroidism shows prolonged jaundice and lethargy.
SubChapter: Metabolic & Hematologic Disorders

Q749. Answer: A

Explanation: Neonatal abstinence syndrome requires a low-stimulation environment to reduce stress and seizures. Gentle swaddling and minimizing noise promote regulation. Handling increases irritability, and feeding should continue carefully to meet caloric needs. Phototherapy is unrelated unless jaundice develops.
SubChapter: Neurologic & Thermoregulatory Disorders

Q750. Answer: A

Explanation: Conjugated hyperbilirubinemia with pale stools and dark urine indicates biliary atresia, a condition of bile duct obstruction. It leads to progressive liver failure if untreated. Physiologic and breast milk jaundice cause unconjugated elevation, while hemolysis produces anemia and early-onset jaundice.
SubChapter: Metabolic & Hematologic Disorders

Made in United States
Orlando, FL
04 November 2026

90206042R00111